BEYOND RELIEF

The DMSO Handbook for Natural Healing, Pain & Inflammation Control with Practical Protocols

Linden Hayes

1

Table of Content

Chapter 1:
Introduction to DMSO and Health Benefits

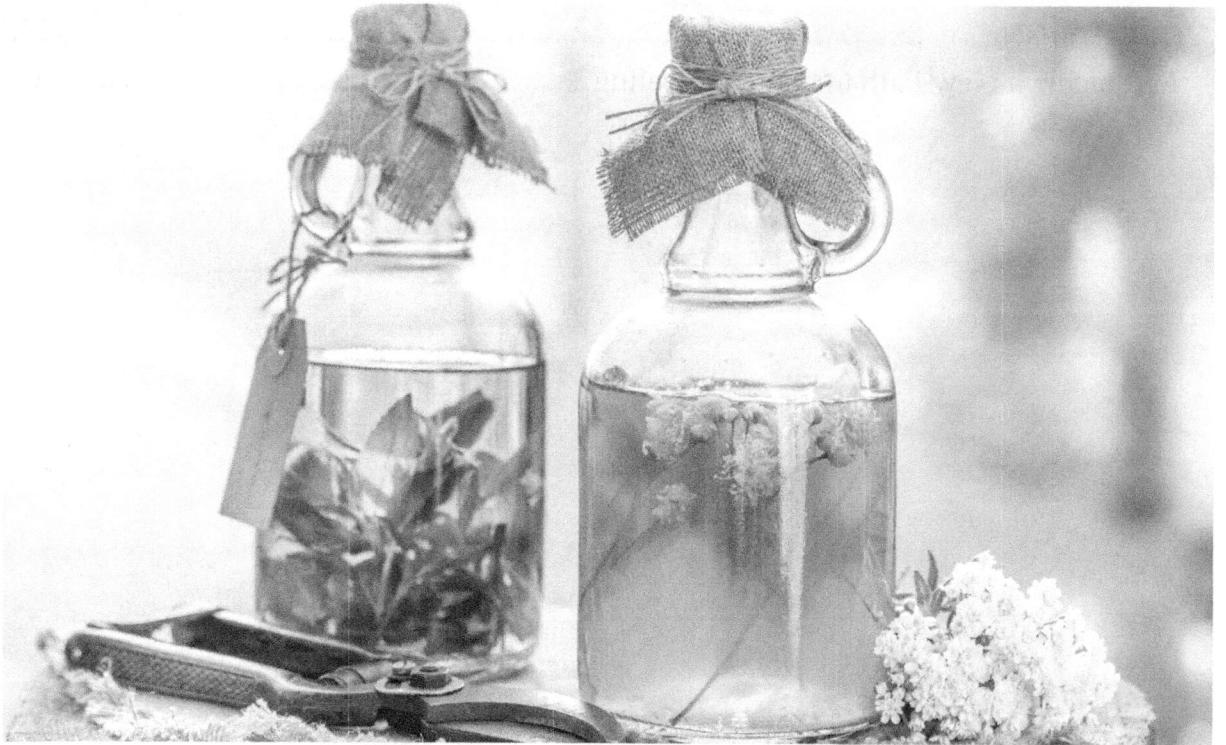

DMSO, or dimethyl sulfoxide, is a compound that has captured the attention of the natural healing community due to its remarkable ability to penetrate the skin and other biological membranes without causing damage. Its discovery in the mid-20th century opened the doors to a myriad of potential health benefits, particularly in the realm of pain management and inflammation reduction. Unlike conventional treatments that often come with a host of side effects, DMSO offers a gentler approach, aligning with the body's natural healing processes. This unique compound has been the subject of extensive research, revealing its capabilities not only as a penetrant but also as an anti-inflammatory agent, an antioxidant, and a cell protector. These properties make DMSO an invaluable tool in the natural health practitioner's arsenal, offering hope to those seeking alternatives to traditional pharmaceuticals.

The versatility of DMSO extends beyond its biochemical roles. It serves as a carrier for other therapeutic agents, enhancing their efficacy by facilitating deeper tissue penetration. This synergistic effect allows for lower doses of accompanying medications, potentially reducing the risk of adverse reactions. Furthermore, DMSO's antioxidant properties contribute to its ability to neutralize free radicals, thereby protecting cells from damage and supporting the body's overall resilience against stress and disease.

Despite its promising benefits, the use of DMSO is not without controversy. Regulatory bodies have been cautious in their endorsement, leading to a landscape where access and information can be fragmented. This has not deterred its growing popularity among those who have experienced its effects firsthand, nor has it dampened the enthusiasm of researchers and clinicians exploring its applications in various medical fields. As the body of evidence supporting DMSO's therapeutic potential continues to expand, so too does the dialogue surrounding its place in both alternative and mainstream medicine.

One of the most compelling aspects of DMSO is its potential to address chronic pain and inflammation, conditions that affect millions worldwide. The mechanisms by which DMSO exerts its pain-relieving and anti-inflammatory effects are multifaceted, involving the modulation of certain biochemical pathways and the reduction of inflammatory markers. For individuals dealing with conditions such as arthritis, fibromyalgia, and other musculoskeletal disorders, DMSO presents a beacon of hope. Its ability to penetrate deeply into tissues makes it particularly effective in reaching areas that topical treatments typically cannot access.

As we delve deeper into the science behind DMSO and its therapeutic applications, it becomes clear that this compound is more than just a simple remedy. It is a testament to the power of natural substances to influence health and well-being in profound ways. The journey to understand and harness the full potential of DMSO is ongoing, with each study and personal testimony adding to the collective knowledge base. For those seeking natural solutions to their health challenges, DMSO represents a fascinating and promising avenue of exploration.

Given its potential for profound impact on health, it's crucial for users and practitioners alike to approach DMSO with informed caution. The safety profile of DMSO is generally favorable, especially when used according to established guidelines. However, like any therapeutic agent, it requires respect for its pharmacological potency and an understanding of proper application methods. This includes considerations for concentration, dilution, and the avoidance of contaminants that could be inadvertently carried into the body due to DMSO's penetrating properties.

Education on the correct use of DMSO is paramount. For topical applications, ensuring the skin is clean and free from chemicals or cosmetics is a basic yet vital step. The concentration of DMSO in solutions can vary significantly, from very dilute preparations for sensitive skin areas to more concentrated solutions for deep tissue penetration. The decision on concentration should be guided by the nature of the condition being treated, the area of application, and individual sensitivity. Moreover, the integration of DMSO into a holistic health regimen underscores the importance of a comprehensive approach to wellness. It's not merely about addressing symptoms but fostering an environment within the body that supports healing and resilience. This may involve dietary adjustments, stress management techniques, and the inclusion of other complementary therapies to enhance DMSO's efficacy.

The narrative surrounding DMSO is one of discovery, debate, and ongoing exploration. Its journey from an industrial solvent to a pivotal player in natural healing narratives exemplifies the dynamic nature of health science and the continuous quest for effective, safe, and natural treatment modalities. As research progresses, the potential for DMSO to play a significant role in managing not only pain and inflammation but also in promoting cellular health, reducing oxidative stress, and supporting the immune system becomes increasingly apparent.

Engagement with the medical community and adherence to regulatory guidance remain critical as the use of DMSO evolves. For those navigating the complexities of chronic conditions, DMSO offers a ray of hope and an invitation to explore the synergies between nature and science. The empowerment of individuals to make informed health decisions, armed with knowledge and supported by a community of practitioners and fellow users, is at the heart of the DMSO narrative.

1.1: WHY DMSO? UNDERSTANDING ITS POTENTIAL

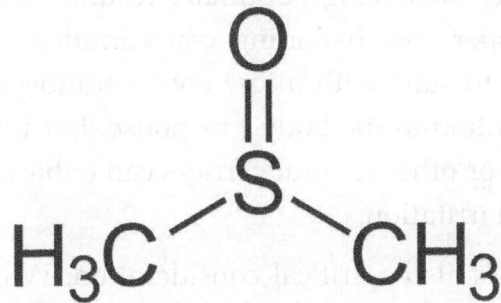

$$O$$
$$\|$$
$$S$$

$$H_3C \qquad CH_3$$

DMSO's unique potential lies in its **molecular structure**, which allows it to **penetrate the skin** and other biological barriers with unparalleled efficiency. This characteristic is what sets DMSO apart from other therapeutic agents, enabling it to deliver relief directly to affected areas. The compound's ability to act as a **carrier** enhances the effectiveness of other medications by facilitating their deeper penetration into tissues. This can be particularly beneficial in treating **localized pain** and **inflammation**, where targeted action is required. Moreover, DMSO's **anti-inflammatory** properties are significant. It works by modulating the body's inflammatory responses, thereby reducing swelling and pain at the source. This is not merely a superficial effect; DMSO influences cellular processes that are fundamental to the inflammatory response, offering a natural and potent means of managing conditions characterized by chronic inflammation.

Another aspect of DMSO's potential is its role as an **antioxidant**. By scavenging harmful free radicals, DMSO protects cells from oxidative stress, a key factor in aging and many diseases. This antioxidant action complements its anti-inflammatory effects, contributing to its overall therapeutic value. The compound's protective effect on cells extends to its ability to stabilize cell membranes, safeguarding them from damage that could lead to cell death. This property is particularly relevant in the context of injury recovery, where cell integrity is crucial for effective healing.

The versatility of DMSO also includes its **analgesic** properties, offering pain relief without the side effects commonly associated with pharmaceutical painkillers. Its mechanism of action involves blocking nerve conduction fibers that produce pain, providing a non-addictive pain management option. This makes DMSO an attractive choice for those seeking alternatives to conventional pain medication, particularly in the context of chronic pain management.

For individuals exploring natural healing solutions, DMSO presents a compelling option. Its multifaceted therapeutic profile, characterized by anti-inflammatory, antioxidant, and analgesic properties, addresses a broad spectrum of health concerns. From managing acute injuries to providing relief from chronic conditions, DMSO's potential applications are extensive. However, achieving optimal results with DMSO requires an understanding of its proper use, including concentration, dilution, and application techniques. It is essential to start with a low concentration and gradually increase as needed, paying close attention to the body's response. For topical applications, mixing DMSO with aloe vera gel or other natural carriers can enhance its skin-soothing effects and mitigate any potential irritation.

The safety of DMSO use is also a critical consideration. While its profile is generally favorable, users must be mindful of potential side effects, such as skin irritation or dryness. Ensuring the skin is clean and free from contaminants before application is crucial to avoid unwanted reactions. It is also advisable to conduct a patch test before widespread use, especially for individuals with sensitive skin. Incorporating DMSO into a holistic health regimen amplifies its benefits. This includes adopting a healthy diet, staying hydrated, and managing stress, all of which support the body's natural healing processes. For those dealing with chronic conditions, consulting with a healthcare professional before starting DMSO is recommended to ensure it complements existing treatments effectively.

The exploration of DMSO's therapeutic potential is a testament to the growing interest in natural and integrative approaches to health and wellness. As research continues to uncover new applications and refine existing protocols, DMSO remains a subject of fascination and hope for many seeking relief from pain and inflammation. Its role in natural healing is a reminder of the power of nature to offer solutions to some of our most pressing health challenges, highlighting the importance of ongoing inquiry and open-minded exploration in the quest for well-being.

1.2: SAFETY FIRST IN SELF-CARE AND DMSO USE

When considering the use of DMSO for self-care, it's paramount to prioritize safety to ensure that the benefits of this powerful compound are maximized without adverse effects. The first step in safe DMSO application involves choosing the right concentration for your needs. **Dilution** is key, as pure DMSO is potent and may cause skin irritation or dryness. For most topical applications, a solution ranging from **30% to 70% DMSO** in distilled water is recommended. It's crucial to start with a lower concentration, especially if you have sensitive skin, and gradually increase as your tolerance is assessed.

Before applying DMSO, perform a **patch test** by applying a small amount of the diluted solution to a discreet area of your skin. Wait for 24 hours to observe any reactions. This step cannot be overstated, as individual sensitivity to DMSO can vary widely. In the event of redness, itching, or discomfort, reduce the concentration or discontinue use and consult a healthcare professional.

The application site should be **clean and free from any other substances**, as DMSO's penetrating properties can carry compounds from the skin's surface into the body. This means avoiding application areas where lotions, creams, or perfumes have been recently applied. Additionally, ensure your hands and the application area are washed with soap and water to remove any residues that could be transported by DMSO into the body.

Using **gloves** or a **clean applicator** such as a cotton ball or pad is advisable to avoid transferring unwanted substances from your hands. Apply the DMSO solution gently to the affected area, allowing it to air dry without covering it immediately with clothing or bandages, as these could absorb the DMSO and affect its efficacy or lead to skin irritation.

Storage of DMSO should be in a **cool, dark place** to maintain its stability. DMSO can degrade over time if exposed to high temperatures or direct sunlight, which can affect its safety and effectiveness. Ensure the container is tightly sealed to prevent contamination and evaporation.

For those considering DMSO for conditions beyond minor aches and pains, such as chronic inflammatory conditions or more severe injuries, **consultation with a healthcare professional** is strongly recommended. This ensures that DMSO use is appropriate for your specific health situation and that it won't interfere with other medications or treatments you may be undergoing. Monitoring your body's response to DMSO is crucial. If you experience persistent irritation, headaches, dizziness, or any other unusual symptoms, discontinue use immediately and seek medical advice. These symptoms could indicate sensitivity to DMSO or an improper application method.

Incorporating DMSO into your self-care regimen requires a commitment to **education** and **caution**. By understanding the proper use of DMSO, including its dilution,

11

application, and potential interactions, you can safely explore the benefits of this remarkable compound. Remember, the goal is to support your body's natural healing processes without causing additional stress or harm. With careful consideration and adherence to safety guidelines, DMSO can be a valuable addition to your natural health toolkit.

Part 1:
Understanding DMSO

Chapter 2:
The Origins and Science Behind DMSO

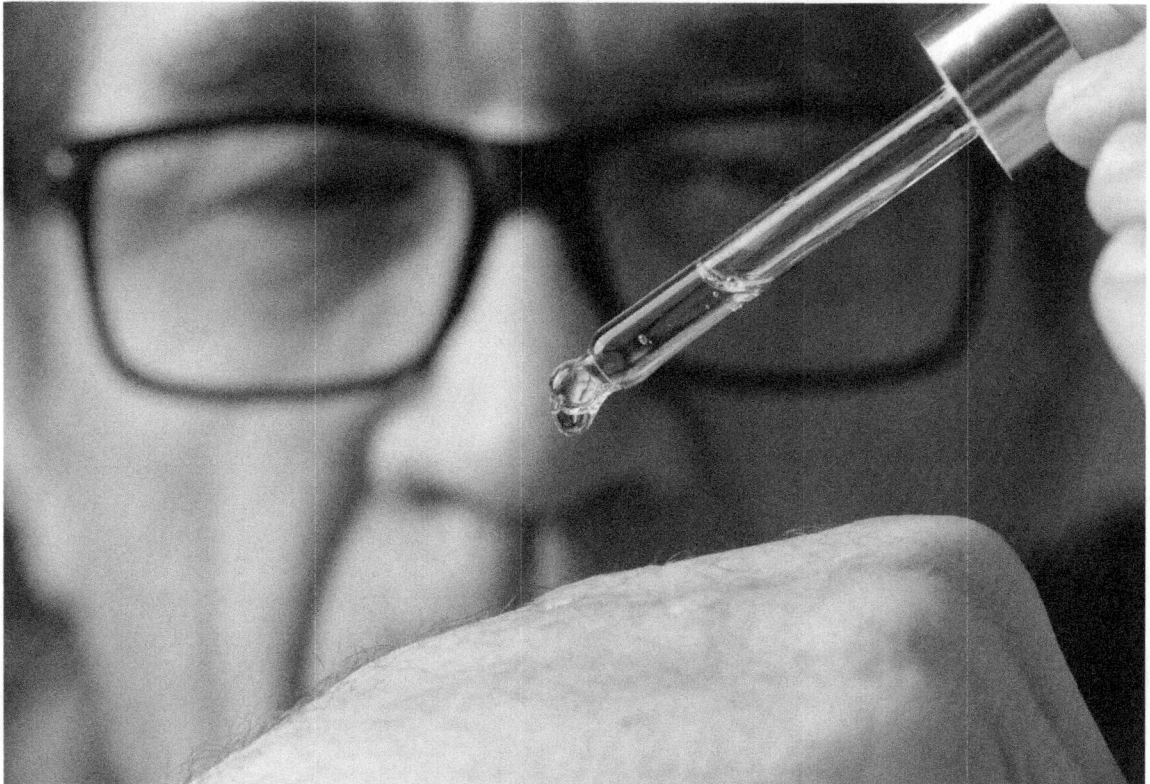

Dimethyl sulfoxide, commonly known as DMSO, has a rich history that dates back to its discovery in 1866 by the Russian scientist Alexander Zaytsev. However, it wasn't until the mid-20th century that DMSO began to gain recognition for its potential therapeutic applications. Initially used as an industrial solvent, the compound's unique ability to penetrate biological membranes without damaging them quickly caught the attention of medical researchers. This characteristic of DMSO opened up new avenues for drug delivery systems, particularly because it could carry other compounds through the skin and into the body, acting as an effective transporter.

The turning point for DMSO came in the 1960s when Dr. Stanley Jacob, a researcher at the University of Oregon, began investigating its potential in medicine. Jacob's work demonstrated that DMSO could reduce inflammation, relieve pain, and preserve living cells from freeze damage. These findings sparked a surge of interest in DMSO's therapeutic benefits, leading to numerous studies and clinical trials aimed at exploring its efficacy in treating a variety of conditions. Despite the promising results in pain management, inflammation control, and even some autoimmune diseases, DMSO's journey towards acceptance in the medical community was met with regulatory hurdles. The FDA's cautious stance on approving DMSO for widespread medical use, citing the need for more comprehensive research to fully understand its pharmacokinetics and potential side effects, limited its availability for therapeutic applications.

Nevertheless, the interest in DMSO did not wane. The compound's anti-inflammatory and analgesic properties continued to be leveraged in veterinary medicine, where it was used to treat musculoskeletal conditions in large animals, such as horses. This veterinary application of DMSO provided further anecdotal evidence of its effectiveness, which, in turn, fueled ongoing research into its mechanisms of action.

One of the most intriguing aspects of DMSO is its dual role as both a pharmaceutical agent and a solvent. Its ability to dissolve both polar and nonpolar compounds makes it exceptionally versatile in research and industry. However, it is this same property that necessitates careful consideration when used therapeutically, as DMSO can carry other substances through the skin and into the bloodstream. Understanding the chemical properties of DMSO, including its molecular structure that facilitates this deep penetration, is crucial for harnessing its therapeutic potential while minimizing risks.

The scientific exploration of DMSO has revealed its impact on cellular processes, particularly its interaction with membranes and proteins. Studies have shown that DMSO can alter the fluidity of cellular membranes, affecting the function of membrane-bound proteins and receptors. This action at the cellular level could explain some of DMSO's therapeutic effects, such as reducing inflammation by modulating the activity of inflammatory cytokines. Moreover, DMSO's role as an antioxidant, scavenging harmful free radicals, adds another layer to its multifaceted therapeutic profile. These antioxidative properties further contribute to its potential in managing conditions associated with oxidative stress.

Despite the challenges in fully integrating DMSO into mainstream medical practice, its use in alternative and complementary medicine continues to grow. The compound's ability to address a wide range of health issues, from acute injuries to chronic conditions, without the severe side effects often associated with pharmaceutical drugs, makes it an appealing option for those seeking natural healing solutions. As research progresses, the scientific community is gradually uncovering the complexities of DMSO's actions in the body, providing a stronger foundation for its therapeutic use.

The exploration of DMSO's pharmacological effects extends beyond its anti-inflammatory and analgesic properties, delving into its potential as a cytoprotective agent. This aspect of DMSO's action is particularly significant in the context of cryopreservation, where it has been utilized to protect cells from ice crystal formation during freezing. The ability of DMSO to penetrate cell membranes without causing damage is a critical factor in its effectiveness in preserving the integrity of cellular structures under extreme conditions. This property not only underscores DMSO's versatility as a therapeutic agent but also highlights its role in biomedical research and tissue preservation.

In addition to its direct effects on cells and tissues, DMSO has been studied for its immunomodulatory capabilities. Preliminary research suggests that DMSO may influence the immune system in a manner that could be beneficial for managing autoimmune diseases and reducing the severity of allergic reactions. These findings open new avenues for the use of DMSO in treating complex immune-related conditions, further expanding its potential therapeutic applications.

The safety profile of DMSO, while generally favorable, requires careful consideration of its pharmacokinetics and interactions with other substances. The compound's ability to enhance the absorption of topical medications raises important considerations for its use in combination therapies. Ensuring that DMSO is used in a controlled manner, with attention to concentration and the nature of substances it is combined with, is paramount to maximizing its therapeutic benefits while minimizing potential risks.

The regulatory landscape for DMSO continues to evolve as new research sheds light on its pharmacological properties and therapeutic potential. While the FDA has approved DMSO for limited clinical applications, such as the treatment of interstitial cystitis, the compound's broader acceptance in medicine hinges on the outcomes of ongoing and future studies. These studies aim to provide a more comprehensive understanding of DMSO's mechanisms of action, optimal dosing regimens, and long-term safety profile.

The growing interest in natural and holistic approaches to health care has contributed to the resurgence of DMSO as a topic of both scientific inquiry and public interest. Individuals seeking alternative treatments for pain, inflammation, and a variety of other conditions are increasingly exploring DMSO as a potential option. This trend is supported by a wealth of anecdotal evidence, coupled with a growing body of scientific research that seeks to validate and explain the therapeutic effects observed.

For health practitioners and patients alike, the key to harnessing DMSO's potential lies in education and informed use. Understanding the nuances of DMSO's actions within the body, the importance of purity and concentration in its application, and the need for caution when combining it with other treatments is essential. As the scientific community continues to explore the full spectrum of DMSO's therapeutic applications, the compound's role in medicine may well expand, offering new hope for many challenging conditions.

The dialogue surrounding DMSO is characterized by a blend of scientific curiosity, clinical pragmatism, and patient-driven interest. This dynamic interplay of perspectives is driving the ongoing exploration of DMSO's possibilities, with each discovery adding to the collective understanding of its value in health and healing. As research advances, DMSO remains a symbol of the broader quest for effective, safe, and natural remedies that align with the body's own healing mechanisms, embodying the spirit of innovation and resilience that defines the field of natural health solutions.

2.1: DISCOVERY OF DMSO IN HEALTH CARE

The initial discovery of DMSO in the health care sector marked a pivotal moment, transforming it from an industrial solvent to a potential medical marvel. The journey began earnestly in the 1960s when Dr. Stanley Jacob, alongside other researchers at the University of Oregon, identified the compound's profound ability to penetrate the skin without causing damage, a characteristic that set the stage for its medical applications. Their research unveiled DMSO's anti-inflammatory and analgesic properties, which showed promise in treating a variety of conditions, including arthritis, acute injuries, and even certain dermatological issues. This discovery was not just about finding a new drug; it was about unveiling a new way to deliver medications directly to affected areas, potentially revolutionizing how treatments could be administered.

The intrigue around DMSO grew as further studies highlighted its role in preserving tissues from freeze damage, suggesting its use in cryopreservation. This was particularly significant in the field of organ transplantation and cellular research, where maintaining the viability of specimens is crucial. The ability of DMSO to protect cells from ice crystal formation during freezing opened new avenues in biomedical research, offering a glimpse into its versatile applications beyond pain management.

Despite the burgeoning interest and the accumulating evidence of its benefits, DMSO's journey was met with skepticism and regulatory challenges. The FDA's hesitance to approve DMSO for broad medical use stemmed from concerns over its safety profile and the need for more comprehensive research to understand its effects fully. This caution was partly due to DMSO's solvent properties, which allow it to carry other substances through the skin and into the bloodstream, raising questions about potential unintended consequences when used as a carrier for other medications.

The regulatory hurdles did not, however, dampen the enthusiasm among those who had experienced DMSO's benefits firsthand. Many individuals turned to DMSO for relief from chronic pain and inflammation, often as a last resort after conventional treatments had failed. This grassroots level of support helped sustain interest in DMSO, even as the medical community grappled with its official stance on the compound.

Veterinary medicine became an unexpected beneficiary of DMSO's therapeutic properties, where it was used extensively to treat musculoskeletal conditions in animals. The success of DMSO in veterinary applications provided compelling anecdotal evidence of its efficacy, further fueling the desire among researchers and clinicians to explore its potential in human medicine.

The journey of DMSO from an obscure industrial solvent to a compound of medical interest is a testament to the serendipitous nature of scientific discovery. It underscores the importance of keeping an open mind and pursuing research even when the path forward is fraught with uncertainty. The story of DMSO is far from over, with ongoing studies aiming to unlock its full therapeutic potential and navigate the regulatory landscape to bring its benefits to a wider audience.

As DMSO continues to be explored in various medical and scientific contexts, its potential to contribute to health and healing remains significant. The key to unlocking this potential lies in rigorous research, thoughtful consideration of its pharmacological properties, and a commitment to understanding how best to harness its capabilities for the greater good. The journey of DMSO in health care is a compelling narrative of innovation, challenge, and the relentless pursuit of solutions that can improve lives.

2.2: UNIQUE CHEMICAL PROPERTIES OF DMSO

DMSO, or dimethyl sulfoxide, possesses a unique chemical structure that sets it apart from other therapeutic compounds. Its molecule consists of two methyl groups attached to a sulfur atom, which is in turn bonded to an oxygen atom. This configuration grants DMSO a highly polar nature, enabling it to dissolve both polar and nonpolar compounds with ease. This solubility spectrum is rare among solvents, making DMSO exceptionally versatile in medical and pharmaceutical applications. The ability to dissolve a wide range of substances allows DMSO to act as a carrier or delivery system for drugs, enhancing their absorption through biological membranes, including the skin and gastrointestinal tract.

DMSO's penetrating ability is perhaps its most renowned feature. It can traverse the skin and other cellular membranes without causing structural damage, a property attributed to its small molecular size and polar nature. This characteristic is crucial for topical applications, where DMSO facilitates the deep tissue delivery of therapeutic agents. When applied to the skin, DMSO interacts with the lipid molecules in the cell membranes, temporarily altering their structure to increase permeability. This effect, however, is reversible and does not harm the cells, making DMSO a safe and effective penetration enhancer.

Anti-inflammatory and analgesic properties of DMSO also contribute to its uniqueness. It modulates inflammation by scavenging hydroxyl radicals and inhibiting the transmission of pain signals through nerve fibers. These actions make DMSO an invaluable tool in managing pain and inflammation, offering relief in conditions such as arthritis, muscle injuries, and burns. The compound's ability to reduce swelling and alleviate pain without the side effects commonly associated with NSAIDs and opioids is a significant advantage, highlighting its potential as a natural therapeutic agent.

Antioxidant capabilities further distinguish DMSO. By neutralizing free radicals, DMSO protects cells from oxidative stress, which is implicated in aging and various diseases. This antioxidative action complements its anti-inflammatory effects, contributing to its overall therapeutic value. The protective effect on cells extends to its ability to stabilize cell membranes, safeguarding them from damage that could lead to cell death. This property is particularly relevant in the context of injury recovery, where cell integrity is crucial for effective healing.

The **immunomodulatory effects** of DMSO are an area of growing interest. Preliminary research suggests that DMSO may influence the immune system in ways that could be beneficial for managing autoimmune diseases and reducing the severity of allergic reactions. These findings open new avenues for the use of DMSO in treating complex immune-related conditions, further expanding its potential therapeutic applications.

In terms of **safety and pharmacokinetics**, DMSO's profile is generally favorable. It is metabolized in the human body to dimethyl sulfide, a compound excreted through the breath and skin, which is responsible for the characteristic garlic-like odor associated with DMSO use. The compound's low toxicity and ability to be excreted from the body underscore its suitability for therapeutic use, provided it is applied judiciously and in appropriate concentrations.

For those considering DMSO for therapeutic applications, it is essential to use pharmaceutical-grade DMSO to ensure purity and safety. The concentration of DMSO in formulations should be carefully selected based on the intended use, with lower concentrations (e.g., 30-70%) typically used for topical applications to minimize the risk of skin irritation. When preparing DMSO solutions, it is crucial to use distilled water or other solvents that are free from contaminants, as DMSO's penetrating properties can carry impurities into the body, potentially leading to adverse effects.

The unique chemical properties of DMSO, including its solubility, penetrating ability, anti-inflammatory and analgesic effects, antioxidant capabilities, and safety profile, make it a compound of significant interest in natural healing and medicine. Its versatility and broad therapeutic potential continue to inspire research and application in various medical fields, offering hope for individuals seeking alternative and complementary treatments for a wide range of conditions.

Chapter 3:
How DMSO Works in the Body

3.1: ABSORPTION AND CELLULAR PENETRATION

DMSO's remarkable ability to penetrate the skin and cellular membranes is a cornerstone of its therapeutic utility, facilitating the delivery of various compounds into the body. This unique characteristic is attributed to its small molecular size and the polarity that allows it to dissolve in both aqueous and lipid environments, making it an ideal vehicle for transdermal drug delivery. When applying DMSO, it's crucial to ensure the skin area is clean and free from any contaminants. Given DMSO's potent carrier properties, any substance present on the skin can potentially be transported into the bloodstream, emphasizing the importance of using pharmaceutical-grade DMSO and adhering to strict hygiene practices.

For effective absorption, DMSO should be applied in a well-ventilated area to prevent inhalation of vapors, which can be irritating to the respiratory tract. Using gloves made of materials resistant to DMSO, such as nitrile, is advisable to avoid unintentional skin contact. When diluting DMSO for application, distilled water or another solvent compatible with DMSO and safe for human consumption should be used to ensure the solution's purity and safety. The concentration of DMSO in the solution plays a pivotal role in its penetration ability and therapeutic effectiveness, with lower concentrations generally recommended for initial use to gauge individual tolerance.

The application method significantly influences DMSO's absorption and distribution within the body. Techniques such as gentle massage can enhance penetration, but care must be taken to apply minimal pressure to avoid skin irritation. For targeted delivery, DMSO can be mixed with specific therapeutic agents, considering the solubility and stability of the agent in DMSO. This combination should be prepared immediately before use to maintain the potency of the active ingredients.

Temperature impacts DMSO's viscosity and, consequently, its absorption rate. Warming the solution to body temperature can facilitate smoother application and faster skin penetration. However, it's essential to avoid using heat sources that could degrade DMSO or the co-administered compound. After application, covering the area with breathable, non-absorbent material may protect clothing and furniture from stains without hindering the absorption process.

Monitoring the response to DMSO application is crucial for adjusting concentration and application frequency. Initial applications should be observed for any adverse reactions, such as skin irritation or allergic responses, and the regimen adjusted accordingly.

Documenting the effects, both positive and negative, can provide valuable insights into the optimal use of DMSO for individual needs.

Incorporating DMSO into a holistic health strategy requires understanding its mechanisms and respecting its potent ability to carry substances into the body. By following these guidelines for safe and effective application, individuals can leverage DMSO's unique properties for enhanced therapeutic outcomes. Engaging with healthcare professionals knowledgeable about DMSO can provide additional support and guidance tailored to personal health objectives, ensuring that its use is both beneficial and safe.

3.2: ANTI-INFLAMMATORY MECHANISMS

DMSO's anti-inflammatory mechanisms are a cornerstone of its therapeutic benefits, particularly in the management of pain and inflammation. The compound's ability to inhibit the migration of leukocytes to the site of injury minimizes the cellular response that leads to inflammation. This action not only reduces swelling but also alleviates the pain associated with inflammation. By targeting the leukocytes, DMSO directly impacts one of the body's primary responses to injury, offering a natural and effective means of controlling inflammation without the use of synthetic drugs that often come with a host of side effects.

Furthermore, DMSO's interaction with hydroxyl radicals plays a significant role in its anti-inflammatory effects. Hydroxyl radicals are highly reactive molecules that can cause significant damage to cells and tissues, exacerbating inflammation and delaying healing. DMSO's ability to scavenge these radicals helps to mitigate their harmful effects, thereby reducing oxidative stress and promoting a more conducive environment for healing. This antioxidant property of DMSO is particularly beneficial in chronic inflammatory conditions where oxidative stress is a persistent problem.

In addition to its direct anti-inflammatory actions, DMSO enhances the body's natural repair processes. It promotes fibroblast proliferation, which is crucial for tissue repair and regeneration. Fibroblasts are cells that play a critical role in wound healing, producing collagen and other extracellular matrix components that are necessary for tissue strength and integrity. By stimulating fibroblast activity, DMSO not only aids in reducing inflammation but also accelerates the healing process, making it an invaluable tool in the management of both acute injuries and chronic conditions.

DMSO's role in modulating the immune response further underscores its potential in treating autoimmune and inflammatory disorders. It has been observed to reduce excessive inflammatory reactions without compromising the body's defense mechanisms. This delicate balance is crucial in autoimmune conditions where the immune system mistakenly attacks the body's own tissues, leading to chronic inflammation and tissue damage. DMSO's ability to modulate these responses can help in managing symptoms and improving the quality of life for individuals with these conditions.

The application of DMSO in transdermal drug delivery systems highlights its versatility as a therapeutic agent. Its solvent properties allow for the creation of topical formulations that can deliver medications directly to the site of pain or inflammation, offering localized treatment without the systemic side effects associated with oral medications. This method of delivery is particularly advantageous for drugs that are poorly absorbed orally or that undergo significant degradation in the digestive system. By bypassing the gastrointestinal tract, DMSO-based transdermal systems ensure that a higher concentration of the active drug reaches the target tissue, enhancing efficacy and reducing the risk of adverse effects.

For individuals considering DMSO as part of their health regimen, it is imperative to prioritize the use of pharmaceutical-grade DMSO to ensure purity and safety. The concentration of DMSO in topical formulations should be carefully selected based on the specific condition being treated and the individual's sensitivity to the compound. Starting with a lower concentration and gradually increasing it can help in identifying the optimal dose that provides therapeutic benefits without causing irritation or other side effects. It is also essential to apply DMSO to clean, intact skin to prevent the introduction of contaminants into the bloodstream and to avoid covering the treated area with occlusive dressings that could enhance absorption beyond desired levels.

Engaging with a healthcare professional knowledgeable about DMSO is crucial for anyone looking to incorporate it into their treatment plan. A healthcare provider can offer guidance on the appropriate use of DMSO, including potential interactions with other medications and how to monitor for adverse effects. This collaborative approach ensures that the use of DMSO is tailored to the individual's needs, maximizing its therapeutic potential while minimizing risks.

3.3: DMSO AS ANTIOXIDANT AND CELL PROTECTOR

DMSO's role as an **antioxidant** and **cell protector** is pivotal in its therapeutic applications, particularly in mitigating oxidative stress, a condition characterized by an imbalance between free radicals and antioxidants in your body. Free radicals are oxygen-containing molecules with an uneven number of electrons, allowing them to easily react with other molecules. These reactions can cause large chain chemical reactions in your body because they react so easily with other molecules. These reactions are called oxidation. They can be beneficial or harmful. Antioxidants are substances that can prevent or slow damage to cells caused by free radicals, unstable molecules that the body produces as a response to environmental and other pressures. The body has its own antioxidant defenses to keep free radicals in check. However, factors such as pollution, radiation, cigarette smoke, and herbicides can also spawn free radicals. If the body cannot process and remove free radicals efficiently, oxidative stress can result. This can harm cells and body function. Oxidative stress is linked to heart disease, cancer, arthritis, stroke, respiratory diseases, immune deficiency, emphysema, Parkinson's disease, and other inflammatory or ischemic conditions. DMSO, with its unique chemical structure, scavenges these harmful free radicals, particularly hydroxyl radicals, thereby protecting the cellular components from damage. This antioxidant action is crucial in preventing the onset of diseases linked to oxidative stress, including cardiovascular diseases, neurodegenerative disorders, and various forms of cancer.

Moreover, DMSO's ability to protect cells extends to its role in enhancing the body's natural antioxidant systems. It upregulates the expression of glutathione, one of the most potent intracellular antioxidants. Glutathione plays a significant role in detoxifying harmful substances in the liver, protecting against oxidative damage, and maintaining the immune system's function. By boosting glutathione levels, DMSO not only augments the body's defense mechanism against oxidative stress but also aids in the detoxification process, contributing to overall health and well-being.

The protective effects of DMSO against cellular damage are not limited to its antioxidant properties. DMSO has been shown to stabilize cell membranes, making them less susceptible to damage and permeation by harmful substances. This membrane-stabilizing effect is particularly beneficial in conditions where cell integrity is compromised, such as in cases of traumatic injury, burns, and certain neurological disorders. By maintaining cell membrane integrity, DMSO helps to preserve cellular function and prevent the loss of essential cellular components.

In addition to its direct protective effects on cells, DMSO's role as a cell protector is evident in its ability to modulate the immune response. It has been observed to reduce excessive inflammatory reactions, which can lead to cellular damage and contribute to the progression of chronic diseases. This immunomodulatory effect, combined with its antioxidant and membrane-stabilizing properties, underscores DMSO's potential as a therapeutic agent in managing a wide range of health conditions characterized by inflammation, oxidative stress, and immune dysregulation.

When considering the application of DMSO for its antioxidant and cell-protective benefits, it is essential to use pharmaceutical-grade DMSO to ensure purity and safety. The concentration and method of application should be carefully selected based on the specific condition being treated and the individual's sensitivity to DMSO. Starting with a lower concentration and gradually increasing it can help in identifying the optimal dose that provides therapeutic benefits without causing irritation or other side effects. Furthermore, applying DMSO to clean, intact skin is crucial to prevent the introduction of contaminants into the bloodstream and to maximize its therapeutic effects.

Engaging with a healthcare professional knowledgeable about DMSO is crucial for anyone looking to incorporate it into their treatment plan. A healthcare provider can offer guidance on the appropriate use of DMSO, including potential interactions with other medications and how to monitor for adverse effects. This collaborative approach ensures that the use of DMSO is tailored to the individual's needs, maximizing its therapeutic potential while minimizing risks.

Chapter 4:
Safety and Precautions

4.1: ESSENTIAL SAFETY GUIDELINES FOR DMSO USE

DMSO (dimethyl sulfoxide) is a **powerful and versatile therapeutic compound** that, when used correctly, offers significant benefits for pain relief, inflammation control, and tissue healing. However, due to its unique ability to penetrate the skin and carry substances directly into the bloodstream, proper handling and application are essential to ensure both safety and effectiveness.

By following a few **key safety guidelines**, you can maximize the benefits of DMSO while minimizing any potential risks.

Choosing the Right DMSO

Not all DMSO products are created equal. To ensure safe use, always opt for **pharmaceutical-grade DMSO**, which guarantees purity and suitability for medical applications. **Industrial-grade DMSO**, often used in solvents and manufacturing, may contain impurities that are not safe for topical or internal use.

- Look for **99.9% pure DMSO** labeled as **pharmaceutical or laboratory grade**.
- Avoid products that are **stored in plastic containers**, as DMSO can dissolve certain plastics and introduce contaminants into the solution. **Glass containers are ideal for storage.**

Proper Dilution for Safe Application

DMSO is typically sold in concentrated form and should be **diluted before application**, especially for individuals new to its use. The appropriate dilution depends on the intended purpose and skin sensitivity:

- **For general use (pain relief, inflammation, joint health)** → Start with a **50% solution** (1 part DMSO, 1 part distilled water).
- **For sensitive skin areas (face, neck, thin skin regions)** → Use a **30%-50% solution** to reduce irritation.
- **For stronger applications (deep tissue penetration, severe pain relief)** → A **70% solution** may be used, but should be introduced gradually.

If you are new to DMSO, it is advisable to **start with a lower concentration** and increase gradually based on tolerance.

Safe Application Methods

To ensure safe and effective use, **apply DMSO using clean and sterile materials** to prevent contamination:

1. **Clean the skin thoroughly**
   - Wash the application area with **mild soap and warm water** to remove any dirt, lotions, or chemicals.
   - Dry the area completely before applying DMSO.

2. **Use a sterile applicator**
   - Apply DMSO using **a glass dropper, a clean cotton pad, or sterile gauze**.
   - **Avoid using bare hands** to prevent unwanted substances from being absorbed along with the DMSO.

3. **Allow for proper absorption**
   - Let DMSO sit on the skin for **20 to 30 minutes**, then rinse the area with clean water to remove any residue.
   - Avoid covering the treated area with synthetic fabrics immediately after application.

Minimizing Skin Irritation and Sensitivity

Some individuals may experience **mild redness, tingling, or dryness** when using DMSO, especially at higher concentrations. These effects are typically temporary and can be minimized by:

- **Using a lower concentration** (start with 30%-50% and adjust based on tolerance).
- **Applying a soothing agent after use** (such as **aloe vera, vitamin E oil, or jojoba oil**) to keep the skin hydrated.
- **Rotating application sites** to prevent localized irritation from frequent use.

If irritation persists, dilute the DMSO further and **reduce the frequency of application**.

Ventilation and Storage Considerations

While DMSO is safe when used properly, **some individuals may find its fumes irritating** when applied in enclosed spaces. To minimize discomfort:

- Apply DMSO in a **well-ventilated area** to avoid inhaling any vapors.
- Store in a **cool, dark place** in a tightly sealed **glass container** to maintain potency and prevent contamination.

Avoiding Unintended Absorption of Contaminants

One of DMSO's most distinctive properties is its ability to **carry substances through the skin and into the bloodstream**. While this makes it an effective delivery system for beneficial compounds, it also means that **unwanted chemicals can be absorbed if proper precautions aren't taken**.

To avoid contamination:

- **Ensure the skin is clean** before application—never apply DMSO over **lotions, perfumes, or synthetic chemicals**.

- **Use only purified water for dilution**—tap water may contain impurities that could be carried into the body.

- **Do not mix DMSO with unknown substances** unless their compatibility is confirmed.

Monitoring Your Body's Response

Every individual reacts differently to DMSO, and responses can vary based on skin sensitivity, concentration used, and frequency of application. **Pay close attention to how your body reacts and adjust accordingly**:

- If you experience **persistent irritation**, reduce the concentration or take a break from use.

- If you are taking prescription medications, consult with a healthcare provider to ensure there are no potential interactions.

- If any severe reaction occurs, such as **hives, swelling, or difficulty breathing**, discontinue use and seek medical attention.

Conclusion

DMSO is a **highly effective therapeutic compound** when used correctly, offering significant benefits for pain relief, inflammation control, and tissue healing. By following **proper safety guidelines**, including **choosing high-quality DMSO, using correct dilutions, and ensuring clean application**, you can incorporate it into your wellness routine with confidence.

In the next section, we will explore **how to manage potential side effects** and further optimize your experience with DMSO.

4.2: MANAGING POTENTIAL SIDE EFFECTS

DMSO is widely recognized for its therapeutic benefits, but like any powerful compound, it requires proper handling to minimize potential side effects. While most individuals tolerate DMSO well, some may experience mild reactions, particularly when using it for the first time or at higher concentrations. Understanding how to **identify, prevent, and manage** these effects will allow for a safe and effective experience.

Common Side Effects and How to Address Them

1. **Skin Irritation and Sensitivity**
   o Some users may notice **redness, tingling, or dryness** at the application site. This is typically due to **higher concentrations of DMSO or prolonged contact time**.
   o **Solution:** Start with a **lower concentration (30-50%)**, limit application time to **20-30 minutes**, and apply a **soothing agent** like aloe vera or vitamin E oil after DMSO has dried.

2. **Garlic-Like Taste and Odor**
   o A distinctive **garlic or oyster-like odor** on the breath or skin is a well-documented effect of DMSO's metabolism. It occurs because DMSO breaks down into **dimethyl sulfide (DMS)**, which is exhaled through the lungs and expelled through sweat.
   o **Solution:** While this is harmless, it can be minimized by **staying hydrated, consuming chlorophyll-rich foods, and maintaining good oral hygiene**.

3. **Mild Headaches or Dizziness**
   o A small percentage of users may experience **headaches, dizziness, or lightheadedness**, especially if DMSO is applied in large amounts or in poorly ventilated areas.
   o **Solution:** Ensure **proper ventilation** during application, use **smaller doses initially**, and allow sufficient time between applications to assess tolerance.

4. **Dry or Peeling Skin**
   o Repeated use of DMSO without adequate hydration can lead to **temporary skin dryness or mild peeling**.
   o **Solution:** Apply a **moisturizer (e.g., aloe vera, coconut oil, or jojoba oil)** after absorption to maintain skin hydration.

5. **Digestive Sensitivity (For Oral Use)**

- o Though this book primarily focuses on **topical** DMSO use, some individuals using DMSO orally may experience **nausea or mild digestive discomfort**.
- o **Solution:** If taking DMSO internally, it should always be **properly diluted and consumed on an empty stomach**.

Who Should Be Cautious When Using DMSO?

While DMSO is generally well-tolerated, certain individuals should consult a healthcare professional before using it:

- **Pregnant or breastfeeding women**, due to the ability of DMSO to cross biological membranes.

- **Individuals taking prescription medications**, as DMSO can enhance the absorption and effects of certain drugs.

- **People with severe liver or kidney conditions**, since DMSO is metabolized through these organs.

- **Those with a known allergy to sulfur compounds**, as DMSO is a sulfur-based compound.

Preventing Adverse Reactions: Best Practices

- **Start with a patch test** – Apply a small amount of **diluted** DMSO to a discreet area (e.g., inner forearm) and monitor for **24 hours** before broader application.

- **Use proper dilution** – Higher concentrations are **not always more effective**; many users achieve **excellent results with a 50% solution**.

- **Apply to clean skin** – Avoid using DMSO over **lotions, perfumes, or synthetic substances**, as it can carry these compounds into the body.

- **Monitor frequency of use** – Daily applications are generally safe, but overuse can lead to increased skin sensitivity. **A break of one week after 6-8 weeks of continuous use** is recommended for long-term users.

When to Seek Medical Advice

Although rare, **severe reactions** such as persistent **rash, difficulty breathing, or swelling** may indicate an **allergic response**. In such cases, **discontinue use immediately and consult a healthcare provider**.

Final Considerations

Most side effects associated with DMSO are **mild and temporary**, and **proper use significantly reduces the likelihood of adverse reactions**. By starting with a lower concentration, following best practices, and listening to your body's response, you can **maximize the benefits of DMSO while minimizing any discomfort**.

Part 2:
Getting Started with DMSO

Chapter 5:
Choosing the Right DMSO

5.1: DIFFERENT GRADES OF DMSO

Once you have identified the grade of DMSO most appropriate for your needs, it is equally important to understand how to **verify the purity** and **quality** of the product you are purchasing. This can often be determined by requesting a **Certificate of Analysis (CoA)** from the supplier, which should detail the concentration of DMSO and the presence of any impurities. It is crucial that the CoA confirms the DMSO meets or exceeds the **American Pharmacopeia (USP) standards** for pharmaceutical-grade DMSO, ensuring it is suitable for therapeutic use. For those considering food-grade DMSO, ensure that the product complies with the **Food Chemicals Codex (FCC)** standards, which indicate it is safe for its intended use in food applications.

When it comes to **storing DMSO**, regardless of the grade, it is imperative to use containers made of materials that are resistant to the solvent properties of DMSO. **High-density polyethylene (HDPE)** or **glass containers** are recommended as they do not interact with DMSO, ensuring the stored substance remains pure and effective. It is also advisable to label the container clearly, indicating the concentration of the solution and the date of dilution, if applicable, to avoid any confusion or misuse in the future.

The **application process** for DMSO requires meticulous attention to detail to prevent any adverse effects. Always apply DMSO to **clean, dry skin** to minimize the risk of contaminants being absorbed into the skin along with the DMSO. For those with sensitive skin, a **patch test** is recommended before full application. This involves applying a small amount of DMSO to a discreet area and monitoring for any signs of irritation over 24 hours. If any discomfort, redness, or irritation occurs, it may be necessary to dilute the DMSO further or consult with a healthcare professional before proceeding.

In terms of **dilution**, it is generally recommended to start with a lower concentration of DMSO, particularly for those new to its use. A **50% solution**, prepared by mixing equal parts of DMSO and distilled water, can be a good starting point. This concentration can be adjusted based on individual tolerance and the specific application. It is critical to use **distilled water** for dilution to avoid introducing any impurities that could react with the DMSO or the skin.

Finally, when incorporating DMSO into your health regimen, it is essential to **monitor your body's response** closely. Adjustments to the concentration or frequency of application may be necessary based on your observations. If you experience any persistent discomfort or adverse reactions, it is important to discontinue use and seek professional medical advice. Remember, the goal is to achieve the therapeutic benefits of DMSO safely and effectively, which requires a personalized approach based on your body's unique reactions and the specific health condition being addressed.

5.2: IDENTIFY AND PURCHASE QUALITY DMSO

Identifying and purchasing quality DMSO requires a keen eye and a bit of know-how to ensure you're getting a product that is safe and effective for your needs. It's crucial to start by looking for **pharmaceutical-grade DMSO**, as this grade ensures the highest level of purity and is intended for medical use. This grade of DMSO has been distilled and processed to remove impurities and contaminants that could be harmful or reduce the effectiveness of the product. **Look for labels** that clearly state "pharmaceutical grade" and avoid those that do not specify the grade or seem ambiguous about their sourcing.

Reputable suppliers are your next checkpoint. A trustworthy supplier should provide detailed product information, including the source, grade, and purity level of the DMSO. They should also be transparent about their quality control processes and be willing to provide a **Certificate of Analysis (CoA)** upon request. This document is a testament to the product's compliance with regulatory standards and its purity. It should detail the concentration of DMSO and the absence of harmful impurities. If a supplier cannot or will not provide this information, it may be wise to look elsewhere.

Online reviews and testimonials can offer additional insights into the quality of the product and the reliability of the supplier. While individual experiences can vary, a pattern of positive feedback from users who have purchased and used the DMSO for similar applications as yours can be a good indicator of quality. Conversely, consistent reports of adverse reactions, ineffective results, or poor customer service should raise red flags.

Packaging and storage conditions are also important to consider when purchasing DMSO. Quality DMSO should be packaged in **dark, glass bottles** to protect it from light exposure, which can degrade the product over time. Plastic containers should be avoided as DMSO can leach chemicals from certain plastics, potentially contaminating the solution. Ensure the product is sealed properly to prevent evaporation and contamination.

Price comparison can be tempting, but it's important to remember that extremely low prices might indicate a compromise in quality. While it's wise to look for competitive pricing, products priced significantly below the market rate may not meet the purity and safety standards required for therapeutic use. Investing in a slightly more expensive product from a reputable source can save you from potential health risks and ensure the effectiveness of your DMSO application.

Finally, **customer service** should not be overlooked. A supplier that offers prompt, knowledgeable, and friendly support can be invaluable, especially if you're new to using

DMSO. They should be willing to answer your questions, provide guidance on product use, and assist with any issues that arise during the purchasing process.

By following these guidelines, you can confidently identify and purchase quality DMSO that meets your therapeutic needs. Remember, the effort you put into selecting the right product can significantly impact the safety and success of your DMSO applications.

Chapter 6:
Preparing and Diluting DMSO

When preparing and diluting DMSO, it's essential to understand the process thoroughly to ensure safety and effectiveness. The first step involves selecting the right concentration of DMSO for your specific needs. Pharmaceutical-grade DMSO is typically available in a 99.9% concentration, which is too potent for direct application on the skin. Therefore, dilution is necessary. The concentration of DMSO in a solution can significantly affect its therapeutic properties and potential side effects. A common approach is to start with a 70% DMSO solution, which means 70% DMSO and 30% water. However, depending on the sensitivity of the skin and the intended use, you might need to adjust this ratio. For more sensitive areas or for those who are new to DMSO, a 50% solution, which is half DMSO and half water, is advisable.

The process of diluting DMSO is straightforward but requires precision and attention to detail. Begin by measuring the appropriate amount of pharmaceutical-grade DMSO using a glass measuring cup or syringe for accuracy. Next, add distilled water to achieve the desired concentration. It's crucial to use distilled water rather than tap water to avoid introducing any impurities or minerals that could react with the DMSO. Stir the mixture gently to ensure it's well combined. This can be done using a glass stirrer or a plastic utensil made of a material that DMSO does not dissolve.

When handling DMSO, always wear gloves, preferably nitrile or neoprene, to prevent skin contact with the concentrated solution. DMSO is known to penetrate the skin rapidly, and while it's being diluted, you want to avoid direct exposure to the concentrated form. Additionally, work in a well-ventilated area to avoid inhaling any fumes that may be released during the mixing process.

After preparing your DMSO solution, it's important to store it correctly to maintain its stability and effectiveness. Transfer the diluted DMSO into a glass bottle with a tight-fitting lid to prevent evaporation and contamination. Label the bottle with the concentration of the solution and the date of dilution for future reference. Store the bottle in a cool, dark place, such as a cupboard or a drawer, away from direct sunlight and heat sources.

DMSO's remarkable ability to penetrate the skin makes it an excellent carrier for other therapeutic agents. However, this property also means it can carry substances from the skin's surface into the body. Therefore, ensuring the skin is clean and free from any contaminants or residues before applying DMSO is crucial. Wash the area with mild soap and water, and dry it thoroughly before application.

In summary, the preparation and dilution of DMSO require careful attention to detail to ensure safety and effectiveness. By following these guidelines, you can confidently incorporate DMSO into your health regimen, leveraging its therapeutic benefits while minimizing risks. Remember, individual reactions to DMSO can vary significantly, and what works for one person may not be suitable for another. Personalizing your approach and adjusting based on your experiences and tolerance levels is key to safely incorporating DMSO into your health regimen.

To ensure the highest efficacy and safety of your DMSO solution, it is imperative to adhere to specific guidelines for application and adjustment of concentration based on individual responses. Once you have prepared your DMSO solution, applying it correctly is just as crucial as the preparation process itself. Begin by using a small, clean brush or a cotton swab to apply the solution to the targeted area. This method allows for precise control over the amount used and helps prevent wastage. For larger areas, a clean, lint-free cloth may be soaked in the DMSO solution and gently applied to the skin. It is important to apply the solution evenly, covering the entire area of concern but avoiding oversaturation.

As DMSO is absorbed through the skin, it is vital to monitor the site of application for any signs of irritation or adverse reaction. If redness, itching, or discomfort occurs, it may indicate a need to adjust the concentration of the DMSO solution. In such cases, increasing the amount of distilled water to dilute the solution further can help mitigate these effects. Conversely, if no irritation occurs and the desired therapeutic effects are not achieved, you may consider gradually increasing the concentration of DMSO, always proceeding with caution and closely observing your body's response.

The frequency of application is another factor that may require adjustment. Starting with once daily application is advisable, gradually increasing as needed and tolerated. However, it is crucial to allow at least 24 hours between applications to observe the skin's response and ensure no adverse reactions develop.

For individuals incorporating DMSO into their regimen for the first time, it is essential to start with a conservative approach, both in terms of concentration and frequency of application. This cautious progression allows the body to adjust to DMSO and helps identify the optimal concentration and application schedule for your specific needs.

It is also worth noting that while DMSO can be a powerful tool for natural healing and pain management, it should not be considered a standalone treatment for chronic or severe conditions. Integrating DMSO into a comprehensive health plan, under the guidance of a healthcare professional, can enhance its benefits and ensure a holistic approach to health and wellness.

Incorporating feedback from your body is key to safely and effectively using DMSO. Adjusting the concentration, method of application, and frequency based on personal tolerance and response allows for a customized approach that maximizes benefits while minimizing risks. By following these detailed guidelines and listening to your body, you can harness the therapeutic potential of DMSO as part of a balanced and informed self-care regimen.

6.1: DILUTION GUIDELINES FOR APPLICATIONS

When preparing DMSO solutions for various applications, it's crucial to adhere to specific dilution guidelines to ensure both safety and efficacy. The concentration of DMSO in a solution can significantly affect its therapeutic properties and potential side effects. Here, we provide detailed instructions for creating dilutions at 25%, 50%, 70%, and 90% concentrations, suitable for a range of applications from mild to more intensive treatments.

25% Dilution: Ideal for sensitive skin areas or for individuals new to DMSO therapy. To create a 25% solution, mix one part 99.9% pure DMSO with three parts distilled water. For example, combine 1 ounce of DMSO with 3 ounces of water. This dilution can be used for treating minor inflammations, bruises, or for delicate skin applications.

50% Dilution: This concentration is effective for moderate pain relief and inflammation control. Mix equal parts of DMSO and distilled water to achieve a 50% solution. For instance, blend 2 ounces of DMSO with 2 ounces of water. It's suitable for joint pain, muscle soreness, and mid-level inflammatory conditions.

70% Dilution: A 70% DMSO solution is potent for more severe cases of pain and inflammation. To prepare, mix 7 parts of DMSO with 3 parts water. Using a 10-ounce mixture as an example, combine 7 ounces of DMSO with 3 ounces of water. This concentration can be applied to areas requiring deeper penetration, such as the shoulders, knees, and back.

90% Dilution: Reserved for the most severe and persistent conditions, a 90% solution should be used with caution and under the guidance of a healthcare professional. To create this concentration, mix 9 parts DMSO with 1 part water. In a 10-ounce formulation, this would mean 9 ounces of DMSO to 1 ounce of water. This high concentration is typically used for significant pain relief in cases of acute injury or deep tissue and joint issues.

Important Considerations:

- Always start with the lowest concentration, especially if you are new to DMSO therapy, to assess your skin's sensitivity.

- Use only 99.9% pure DMSO and distilled water to avoid introducing impurities into the solution.

- Conduct a patch test on a small skin area before applying the solution more broadly, especially when using higher concentrations.

- Store DMSO solutions in glass containers to prevent a reaction with plastics.

- Label each solution with the concentration and the date it was made to avoid confusion and ensure proper usage.

By following these guidelines, individuals can safely explore the benefits of DMSO for natural healing, pain, and inflammation control. Remember, the key to effective DMSO therapy lies in starting slow, monitoring your body's response, and adjusting concentrations as needed.

6.2: STEP-BY-STEP DILUTION GUIDE

After establishing the basic dilution percentages and their applications, it's crucial to delve into the practical aspects of creating these solutions with precision and care. The process begins with gathering the necessary materials: a clean, dry glass measuring cup, a glass stir rod, 99.9% pure DMSO, distilled water, and glass storage bottles with tight-fitting lids. It's imperative to use glass equipment to avoid any reaction DMSO might have with plastics or other materials, which could compromise the purity of your solution.

First, measure the appropriate amount of DMSO using the glass measuring cup. For accuracy, ensure the cup is on a level surface and your eye is at the level of the measurement marking. Pour the DMSO slowly to avoid splashing, and check the measurement twice to confirm accuracy. Next, measure the distilled water needed for your dilution. If you're creating a 50% solution, for example, and you've measured 2 ounces of DMSO, you'll then measure 2 ounces of distilled water.

Once both components are measured, pour the distilled water into the container with DMSO. This order helps in reducing the exothermic reaction that occurs when DMSO is mixed with water, which can slightly warm the solution. Use the glass stir rod to mix the solution gently but thoroughly. Stirring should be done carefully to avoid creating bubbles or splashing, as DMSO can be absorbed through the skin upon contact.

After the solution is well mixed, carefully transfer it to a glass storage bottle. Label the bottle with the concentration of the solution and the date it was made. This practice helps in keeping track of the solution's strength and ensures that you are using it within a safe time frame, as the efficacy of DMSO can diminish over time.

For those creating dilutions for the first time or experimenting with a new concentration, conducting a patch test is a critical next step. Apply a small amount of the diluted solution to a discreet area of the skin, preferably somewhere easily monitored for reactions, such as the inside of the wrist. Wait for at least 24 hours to observe any adverse reactions. If irritation, redness, or discomfort occurs, consider reducing the concentration or consulting with a healthcare professional before further application.

In handling DMSO, always wear protective gloves, preferably made of nitrile, to prevent skin absorption during the preparation process. Additionally, work in a well-ventilated area to avoid inhaling any fumes that may be released. DMSO has a distinctive garlic-like odor, which can be noticeable when preparing higher concentration solutions.

Remember, the goal of using DMSO is to aid in healing and pain relief. By taking the time to prepare your solutions with care and precision, you ensure the safest and most effective use of this remarkable compound. Whether you're addressing joint pain, inflammation, or other conditions, the correct dilution of DMSO can be a valuable part of your wellness regimen. Always consult with a healthcare professional if you're unsure about the appropriate concentration for your needs or if you experience any adverse effects. With these guidelines, you're equipped to create DMSO solutions tailored to your therapeutic requirements, ensuring you reap the maximum benefits of your DMSO therapy.

Part 3:
TARGETED DMSO PROTOCOLS FOR PAIN, INFLAMMATION, AND SKIN HEALTH

Chapter 7:
DMSO For Pain Relief – Proven Applications

7.1 THE SCIENCE BEHIND DMSO FOR PAIN MANAGEMENT

Dimethyl sulfoxide (DMSO) is not just another alternative remedy—it's a scientifically validated compound with remarkable pain-relieving properties. Unlike conventional pain medications that merely mask discomfort, DMSO works at a **cellular level**, addressing both the **cause** of pain and the **inflammation** that fuels it.

How DMSO Relieves Pain at the Source

DMSO's ability to penetrate the skin and tissues **within seconds** is what sets it apart. Once absorbed, it travels **deep into muscles, joints, and nerves**, carrying beneficial compounds directly to the affected area. This rapid absorption allows it to:

- **Reduce inflammation:** DMSO inhibits inflammatory cytokines, such as interleukin-6 (IL-6) and tumor necrosis factor-alpha (TNF-α), which are primary drivers of chronic pain conditions like arthritis and fibromyalgia.

- **Block pain signals:** By interacting with pain receptors in the nervous system, DMSO **disrupts pain pathways** at a molecular level, providing lasting relief without the side effects of opioids or NSAIDs.

- **Enhance cellular repair:** As an antioxidant, DMSO neutralizes free radicals and **protects tissues from oxidative stress**, accelerating the healing of damaged muscles, joints, and nerves.

Why DMSO is Different from Conventional Painkillers

Most pain relief medications, including NSAIDs and corticosteroids, work by **temporarily suppressing symptoms**—but they often come with side effects like gastrointestinal issues, liver stress, and dependency risks. DMSO, on the other hand, offers a **safer, non-toxic alternative** that not only relieves pain but also **promotes long-term tissue recovery**.

Additionally, while topical creams and pain patches struggle to penetrate deeper layers of tissue, DMSO **effortlessly crosses biological membranes**, delivering relief exactly where it's needed.

Scientific Backing for DMSO's Pain-Relieving Effects

DMSO's effectiveness is **not just anecdotal** — it has been widely studied in medical and clinical settings. Research has demonstrated its efficacy in treating:

- **Arthritis & joint pain:** Studies show that DMSO significantly reduces stiffness and swelling in osteoarthritis and rheumatoid arthritis patients.

- **Neuropathic pain:** DMSO's neuroprotective properties make it effective for nerve pain, including sciatica and carpal tunnel syndrome.

- **Post-injury recovery:** Athletes and physical therapists have long used DMSO to **speed up muscle recovery** and **reduce soreness** after intense physical exertion.

With its **proven ability to relieve pain, reduce inflammation, and accelerate healing**, DMSO is a **powerful tool for anyone looking for a safe and effective alternative to conventional pain management methods**. In the next section, we'll cover **best practices for applying DMSO safely and effectively** to maximize results.

7.2 HOW TO APPLY DMSO FOR PAIN: BEST PRACTICES AND SAFETY

Using **DMSO correctly** is essential to maximize its pain-relieving benefits while minimizing potential side effects. Unlike conventional topical treatments, **DMSO penetrates the skin and enters the bloodstream almost instantly**, which means it must be handled with care. This section outlines the **best application methods, proper dosages, and safety precautions** to ensure effective and responsible use.

Choosing the Right DMSO Concentration

DMSO is available in various concentrations, typically ranging from **25% to 99% purity**. For pain management, the most commonly used dilutions are:

- **50% to 70% DMSO** – Ideal for joint pain, arthritis, and muscle soreness. This concentration balances effectiveness with skin tolerance.

- **90% DMSO** – Used in some protocols but may cause skin irritation in sensitive individuals. Recommended for **localized, short-term applications** only.

- **25% to 50% DMSO** – Suitable for individuals with sensitive skin or for use on delicate areas like the neck or near joints with thinner skin.

It is always advisable to **start with a lower concentration** and increase gradually based on personal tolerance.

Application Method: Step-by-Step Guide

1. **Clean the Skin Thoroughly**

    o Wash the application area with **mild soap and warm water** to remove any dirt, oil, or residues that could be absorbed along with the DMSO.

    o Pat the skin **completely dry** before applying DMSO.

2. **Use a Clean Applicator**

    o DMSO should be **applied with a glass dropper, a clean cotton pad, or a sterile gauze pad**.

    o Avoid **contaminated materials** (such as plastic applicators or unclean hands) that might introduce impurities into the solution.

3. **Apply a Thin Layer**

    o Use a **small amount** and spread it gently over the affected area.

    o Do not **rub aggressively**—DMSO is absorbed rapidly, and excessive friction can cause irritation.

4. **Allow Proper Absorption Time**

    o Let the solution **fully absorb for 15 to 30 minutes** before covering the area with clothing.

    o Avoid touching the treated area during this time to prevent transferring DMSO to unintended areas.

5. **Rinse Off Residue**

    o After absorption, rinse the skin with **clean water** to remove any excess DMSO.

    o If irritation occurs, **reduce concentration** or apply an aloe vera gel as a skin barrier.

Best Practices for Safe Use

- **Avoid Contact with Contaminants**: DMSO carries substances directly through the skin. Ensure hands and application tools are **completely clean** before use.

- **Limit Frequency**: Start with **one application per day**. If well tolerated, increase to a **maximum of two applications daily** as needed.

- **Rotate Application Sites**: For frequent users, alternating application areas (e.g., knee one day, shoulder the next) can help **minimize skin irritation**.

- **Monitor for Skin Sensitivity**: Mild tingling or warmth is normal. If redness, burning, or itching occurs, dilute the solution further and apply a **moisturizing agent** like aloe vera or vitamin E oil after use.

Who Should Avoid DMSO?

Although DMSO is generally safe when used correctly, certain individuals should **consult a healthcare provider before use**:

- Pregnant or breastfeeding women.

- Individuals taking **blood thinners** or prescription medications (DMSO can enhance absorption and alter drug effects).

- Those with **liver or kidney disorders**, as DMSO is metabolized through these organs.

- People with known **sensitivity to sulfur-based compounds**.

Ensuring Long-Term Safety and Effectiveness

DMSO is a **powerful, research-backed pain relief solution**, but responsible use is crucial. By **following these best practices**, users can maximize its therapeutic potential **without unnecessary risks**. In the next section, we will explore **specific DMSO pain relief protocols for arthritis, back pain, and muscle recovery**—tailored to different conditions and severity levels.

7.3 Targeted Pain Protocols

7.3.1 Joint and Arthritis Relief: Direct DMSO Application and Dosage

Arthritis and joint pain can severely impact mobility and quality of life. Unlike traditional pain relievers, which often provide only temporary relief, **DMSO penetrates deeply into joints, reducing inflammation at its source and promoting long-term relief**. This protocol outlines the correct **application method, dosage, and frequency** for using DMSO to manage arthritis and joint pain effectively.

Why DMSO Works for Joint Pain and Arthritis

DMSO alleviates joint pain by:

Reducing inflammation – It inhibits inflammatory mediators like prostaglandins and cytokines, which contribute to joint stiffness and swelling.

Blocking pain signals – DMSO interacts with nerve fibers to dampen pain perception at the source.

Enhancing circulation – By improving microvascular blood flow, DMSO facilitates nutrient delivery to damaged joint tissues, supporting repair.

Recommended DMSO Concentration for Joint Pain

For **chronic arthritis and joint pain**, the ideal DMSO concentration is **50% to 70%**. Higher concentrations (above 70%) are not necessary and may cause skin irritation.

- **Mild to moderate pain** → Start with a **50% solution** (1 part DMSO, 1 part distilled water).
- **Severe or chronic arthritis** → Use a **70% solution** (7 parts DMSO, 3 parts water).

Application Protocol for Joint Relief

1. Clean the Skin

Wash the affected joint area with warm water and mild soap. Pat dry completely.

2. Apply a Thin Layer of DMSO

Using a sterile cotton pad or gauze, **apply a thin layer of the DMSO solution directly over the painful joint** (knees, hands, shoulders, hips, etc.). Do not rub aggressively — DMSO absorbs rapidly on its own.

3. Allow Absorption

Let the DMSO sit on the skin for **20 to 30 minutes**. Avoid covering the area with clothing during this time to prevent contamination.

4. Rinse Off Residue

After absorption, rinse the skin with **clean water** to remove any remaining DMSO. This step helps reduce irritation and prevents unwanted absorption of contaminants.

Dosage and Frequency

- **Mild pain** → Apply **once daily** for the first week, then adjust as needed.

- **Moderate to severe arthritis** → Apply **twice daily** (morning and evening) for optimal relief.

For long-term arthritis management, use DMSO **for up to six weeks**, then take a break of **one to two weeks** before resuming treatment. This cycle helps prevent skin irritation and maintains effectiveness.

Additional Tips for Enhanced Results

Combine with movement therapy – Gentle stretching or light exercise after application can enhance joint mobility.

Use an anti-inflammatory diet – Reducing processed foods and increasing omega-3 intake supports long-term joint health.

Alternate application sites – If applying DMSO to multiple joints, rotate application sites to minimize skin sensitivity.

DMSO is a **powerful tool for arthritis and joint pain relief**, offering an alternative to pharmaceuticals with **fewer side effects and long-term benefits**. In the next section, we will explore how DMSO can be applied specifically for **back pain and sciatica**, addressing deeper nerve-related discomfort.

7.3.2 Back Pain and Sciatica: How to Maximize Relief

Chronic back pain and sciatica can be debilitating, limiting mobility and diminishing quality of life. Conventional treatments often rely on painkillers or invasive procedures that provide temporary relief but do not address the root cause. **DMSO offers a powerful alternative, penetrating deep into muscle tissue and nerve pathways to reduce inflammation, alleviate nerve compression, and promote long-term healing.**

Why DMSO is Effective for Back Pain and Sciatica

DMSO's ability to **bypass the skin barrier and reach inflamed nerves and muscles** makes it uniquely effective for back pain and sciatic nerve compression. It works by:

- **Reducing inflammation in spinal discs, muscles, and nerves** – This is critical for conditions like herniated discs or degenerative disc disease.

- **Improving circulation in affected areas** – Enhanced blood flow delivers oxygen and nutrients, promoting faster healing of damaged tissues.

- **Interrupting pain signals** – DMSO modulates nerve activity, reducing hypersensitivity and alleviating sciatic nerve pain.

Recommended DMSO Concentration for Back Pain and Sciatica

For **deep tissue penetration and nerve relief**, a **70% DMSO solution** (7 parts DMSO, 3 parts distilled water) is recommended. If skin sensitivity occurs, reduce to **50%**.

Application Protocol for Lower Back and Sciatica Relief

1. **Prepare the Skin**
   - Clean the lower back or affected area with warm water and mild soap.
   - Ensure the skin is completely dry before application.

2. **Apply a Thin Layer of DMSO**
   - Using a **sterile cotton pad or gauze**, apply a thin layer of DMSO **directly over the lower back, spine, or along the sciatic nerve pathway** (from the lower back down the leg).
   - Avoid rubbing aggressively — DMSO will absorb naturally.

3. **Allow Absorption**
   - Let the solution **sit for 20 to 30 minutes** before rinsing the area with water.
   - Do not apply lotions, oils, or creams immediately before or after application.

4. **Repeat as Needed**
   - For mild discomfort, apply **once daily** in the evening.

o   For severe pain, apply **twice daily** (morning and evening).

Best Practices for Maximum Relief

- **Use Heat Therapy After Application** – Applying a **warm compress or heating pad** 15-30 minutes after DMSO absorption can **enhance circulation and relax tight muscles**.

- **Stretch and Move** – Gentle stretching exercises can help **release nerve compression** and improve flexibility.

- **Combine with Magnesium or MSM for Added Benefits** – Magnesium supports muscle relaxation, while MSM (methylsulfonylmethane) enhances the anti-inflammatory effects of DMSO.

When to Expect Results

- **Immediate Relief** – Many users experience **a reduction in pain within the first few applications**.

- **Long-Term Benefits** – Consistent use over **several weeks** can significantly reduce nerve inflammation and chronic pain recurrence.

DMSO's ability to **target deep-seated pain and inflammation makes it a game-changer** for those suffering from persistent back pain and sciatica. In the next section, we will explore **how DMSO can be applied for muscle soreness and injury recovery, ensuring optimal recovery and performance.**

7.3.3 Muscle Soreness and Injury Recovery

Muscle soreness and injuries, whether from intense physical activity, repetitive strain, or accidents, can slow down recovery and impact daily function. Traditional treatments like over-the-counter pain relievers and ice packs provide only temporary relief, while **DMSO works at a deeper level—reducing inflammation, enhancing circulation, and accelerating the body's natural healing process.**

How DMSO Supports Muscle Recovery

DMSO is particularly effective for muscle pain and injuries because of its **rapid absorption and ability to penetrate deep into soft tissues.** It works by:

- **Reducing inflammation and swelling** – DMSO inhibits inflammatory mediators such as prostaglandins, helping to minimize post-exercise soreness and injury-related swelling.

- **Enhancing oxygen and nutrient delivery to muscles** – By improving microcirculation, DMSO accelerates **tissue repair and recovery**.

- **Relieving pain at the source** – Unlike topical pain relievers that mask discomfort, DMSO **blocks pain signals at a cellular level** while promoting healing.

Recommended DMSO Concentration for Muscle Soreness and Injuries

- **For general muscle soreness** → A **50% DMSO solution** (1 part DMSO, 1 part distilled water) is sufficient.

- **For acute injuries or severe muscle strain** → A **70% DMSO solution** (7 parts DMSO, 3 parts distilled water) may be used, but should be tested on a small area first to check for skin sensitivity.

Application Protocol for Muscle Recovery

1. **Clean the Skin**

   o Wash the affected area with warm water and mild soap to remove dirt, sweat, or oils.

   o Pat dry completely before applying DMSO.

2. **Apply a Thin Layer of DMSO**

   o Using a sterile cotton pad or gauze, **apply a thin layer over sore or injured muscles** (legs, arms, shoulders, or any affected area).

   o Do not rub aggressively—allow natural absorption.

3. **Let It Absorb**

   o Leave DMSO on the skin for **20 to 30 minutes** before rinsing with water.

      o Avoid covering the area with tight clothing during this period.

4. **Repeat as Needed**

      o For mild soreness, apply **once daily after exercise or activity**.

      o For injuries, apply **twice daily** (morning and evening) to reduce inflammation and support tissue repair.

Best Practices for Optimal Recovery

- **Apply DMSO Post-Workout** – Using DMSO after exercise can help **reduce delayed onset muscle soreness (DOMS)** and prevent excessive stiffness.

- **Use with Cold Therapy for Acute Injuries** – If applied within the first **24 to 48 hours** of a muscle strain or injury, DMSO can be combined with ice therapy to minimize swelling.

- **Consider Magnesium or MSM for Additional Support** – Combining **DMSO with magnesium oil** can further promote muscle relaxation, while MSM (methylsulfonylmethane) enhances DMSO's anti-inflammatory properties.

Expected Results

- **Immediate Relief** – Many users report a **noticeable reduction in pain and stiffness within the first few applications**.

- **Faster Healing** – Regular use over **one to two weeks** can accelerate the repair of microtears in muscle fibers, speeding up recovery time.

DMSO is a **powerful tool for athletes, fitness enthusiasts, and individuals recovering from injuries**, offering a safe and effective alternative to traditional pain management approaches. In the next section, we will explore its role in **reducing systemic inflammation and supporting long-term wellness.**

Chapter 8:
DMSO for Inflammation Control

8.1 UNDERSTANDING DMSO'S ANTI-INFLAMMATORY MECHANISM

Inflammation is a **natural defense mechanism** — the body's way of responding to injury, infection, or chronic conditions. However, when inflammation becomes excessive or persistent, it can lead to **chronic pain, tissue damage, and degenerative diseases**. Conventional treatments, such as **NSAIDs and corticosteroids**, provide relief but often come with side effects, including gastrointestinal issues and long-term risks to organ health. **DMSO, on the other hand, offers a safer, more targeted approach to inflammation control by working at the cellular level.**

How DMSO Reduces Inflammation

Unlike standard anti-inflammatory drugs that primarily work by blocking pain signals or suppressing immune responses, **DMSO actively targets the biochemical processes that drive inflammation.** Its effectiveness is due to a combination of **unique properties** that allow it to penetrate tissues deeply and modulate inflammatory pathways.

1. Inhibiting Inflammatory Cytokines

DMSO reduces inflammation by **blocking the production of pro-inflammatory cytokines**, including:

- **Tumor Necrosis Factor-alpha (TNF-α)** – A key driver of chronic inflammatory diseases such as arthritis and autoimmune conditions.

- **Interleukin-6 (IL-6) and Interleukin-1 (IL-1)** – Proteins that amplify pain and swelling in response to injury or disease.

By interfering with these inflammatory messengers, **DMSO helps reduce swelling, pain, and tissue degradation**, making it a valuable tool for both acute injuries and chronic inflammatory conditions.

2. Scavenging Free Radicals and Reducing Oxidative Stress

Inflammation is often accompanied by **oxidative stress**, a process in which free radicals damage healthy cells and tissues. DMSO acts as a **potent antioxidant**, neutralizing free radicals before they can cause further harm. This **protects tissues from degeneration** and accelerates recovery from injuries.

3. Enhancing Circulation and Oxygen Delivery

Inflammatory conditions often restrict blood flow to affected areas, **slowing down healing and prolonging pain**. DMSO improves microcirculation, allowing for:

- **Better oxygen delivery to inflamed tissues**
- **More efficient removal of cellular waste and toxins**
- **Faster resolution of swelling and stiffness**

4. Direct Pain Modulation and Nerve Protection

Chronic inflammation often leads to **nerve irritation and heightened pain sensitivity**. DMSO **modulates nerve function**, reducing pain perception while also protecting nerve fibers from inflammation-induced damage.

Why DMSO is a Superior Anti-Inflammatory Option

- **Unlike NSAIDs, DMSO does not harm the stomach lining or kidneys.**
- **Unlike corticosteroids, it does not suppress the immune system or cause systemic side effects.**
- **Unlike topical creams, it penetrates deeply, reaching muscles, joints, and nerves.**

By targeting **inflammation at its source**, DMSO provides **long-term relief** without the risks associated with pharmaceutical anti-inflammatories.

In the next section, we will explore **specific DMSO protocols for managing inflammation**, from acute injuries and post-surgical recovery to chronic inflammatory conditions.

8.2 PROTOCOLS FOR MANAGING INFLAMMATION

8.2.1 Acute Injury and Post-Surgical Recovery

Acute injuries and post-surgical inflammation can significantly delay healing, leading to prolonged pain, swelling, and restricted mobility. Traditional treatments like **NSAIDs and corticosteroids** can provide temporary relief but often come with side effects and may slow tissue repair. **DMSO offers a natural, non-toxic alternative that not only reduces inflammation but also accelerates recovery by enhancing cellular function and circulation.**

Why DMSO Works for Acute Injuries and Surgery Recovery

DMSO is particularly effective for acute injuries and post-surgical care due to its **rapid penetration and ability to modulate inflammation at the source**. It benefits recovery by:

- **Reducing post-surgical swelling and bruising** – DMSO inhibits the inflammatory response that leads to excessive fluid buildup around incisions and injuries.

- **Minimizing scar tissue formation** – By improving collagen remodeling and reducing oxidative stress, DMSO supports more effective tissue regeneration.

- **Enhancing pain relief without medication dependency** – Its ability to block pain signals at a cellular level makes it a valuable alternative to opioids or NSAIDs.

Recommended DMSO Concentration for Acute Injuries and Post-Surgical Sites

For **safe and effective application**, use a **50% DMSO solution** (1 part DMSO, 1 part distilled water). In more severe cases, a **70% solution** can be used, but should be tested first on a small area for skin sensitivity.

Application Protocol for Injury and Surgical Recovery

1. **Clean the Skin Thoroughly**

   o Wash the application area with **mild soap and warm water** to remove contaminants.

   o Dry the area completely before applying DMSO.

2. **Apply a Thin Layer of DMSO**

   o Using a sterile cotton pad or gauze, gently **apply a thin layer over the injured or post-surgical area**.

   o Avoid rubbing aggressively — DMSO absorbs naturally without the need for excessive friction.

3. **Allow Proper Absorption**

  o Let the DMSO sit for **20 to 30 minutes** before rinsing with clean water.

  o Do not apply over **open surgical wounds** — instead, apply around the incision site to reduce inflammation in surrounding tissues.

4. **Repeat as Needed**

  o **For acute injuries**, apply **twice daily** (morning and evening) to control swelling and pain.

  o **For post-surgical recovery**, apply **once daily** during the first week, then increase to **twice daily** if well tolerated.

Best Practices for Enhanced Recovery

- **Pair DMSO with Cold Therapy for Immediate Relief** – Applying ice packs **15-30 minutes after DMSO absorption** can further reduce swelling.

- **Support Collagen Production for Scar Reduction** – Combining DMSO with **vitamin C or aloe vera** can aid tissue repair and reduce post-surgical scarring.

- **Avoid Contaminants During Application** – Always use sterile materials and **avoid lotions, creams, or synthetic fabrics** over the treated area, as DMSO can carry unwanted substances into the bloodstream.

Expected Results

- **First 48 Hours** – Reduction in swelling, improved range of motion, and initial pain relief.

- **1 to 2 Weeks** – Noticeable decrease in inflammation, minimized bruising, and improved healing response.

- **Long-Term** – Enhanced tissue regeneration, reduced scar tissue formation, and more stable recovery.

DMSO's ability to **modulate inflammation, accelerate healing, and reduce post-operative discomfort** makes it an excellent addition to any recovery protocol. In the next section, we will examine **how DMSO can be used for chronic inflammatory conditions such as arthritis, fibromyalgia, and autoimmune disorders.**

8.2.2 Chronic Inflammatory Conditions (Arthritis, Fibromyalgia, Autoimmune)

Chronic inflammation is a **root cause** of many long-term health conditions, including **arthritis, fibromyalgia, and autoimmune disorders**. Unlike acute inflammation, which is a necessary and temporary immune response, chronic inflammation is **persistent and damaging**, leading to **ongoing pain, stiffness, and fatigue**. Standard treatments often rely on **steroids, NSAIDs, or immunosuppressants**, which can come with significant side effects. **DMSO offers a safer, non-toxic alternative that targets inflammation at a cellular level, promoting long-term relief without compromising the immune system.**

How DMSO Helps Manage Chronic Inflammatory Conditions

DMSO is particularly effective in chronic inflammation because of its **deep tissue penetration** and **multi-faceted approach to inflammation control**. It provides relief by:

- **Modulating the Immune Response** – DMSO helps balance **overactive immune activity**, which is a key driver in **autoimmune diseases** such as rheumatoid arthritis, lupus, and multiple sclerosis.

- **Reducing Joint and Muscle Inflammation** – By **blocking pro-inflammatory cytokines**, including **TNF-α and IL-6**, DMSO alleviates swelling, pain, and tissue damage associated with **arthritis and fibromyalgia**.

- **Improving Cellular Oxygenation and Detoxification** – DMSO enhances **oxygen delivery to cells**, improving mitochondrial function and reducing oxidative stress, a major contributor to **chronic pain and fatigue syndromes**.

Recommended DMSO Concentration for Chronic Inflammation

For long-term inflammatory conditions, **a 50% DMSO solution** (1 part DMSO, 1 part distilled water) is generally well tolerated. In more severe cases, a **70% solution** may be used, but should be introduced gradually to assess skin sensitivity.

Application Protocol for Chronic Inflammatory Conditions

1. **Prepare the Skin**
    - Wash the affected area (joints, muscles, or localized pain sites) with **warm water and mild soap** to remove contaminants.
    - Dry thoroughly before applying DMSO.

2. **Apply DMSO to the Targeted Area**
    - Using a sterile cotton pad or gauze, **apply a thin layer of DMSO over the affected joints or muscle regions**.
    - Allow natural absorption—do not rub aggressively.

3. **Let It Absorb and Remove Residue**
   - Leave the solution on the skin for **20 to 30 minutes** before rinsing with clean water.
   - If skin irritation occurs, **reduce the concentration** or apply **aloe vera or vitamin E oil** after absorption to soothe the skin.

4. **Establish a Consistent Routine**
   - **Mild to moderate symptoms** → Apply **once daily** in the evening.
   - **Severe inflammation or flare-ups** → Apply **twice daily** (morning and evening).

For **long-term use,** follow a **six-week cycle,** then take a **one-week break** before resuming treatment. This helps prevent skin irritation while maintaining effectiveness.

Additional Strategies for Enhanced Results

- **Combine with Movement Therapy** – Gentle stretching, yoga, or light resistance exercises can **help maintain joint mobility and prevent stiffness**.

- **Support Mitochondrial Function** – Nutrients such as **magnesium, CoQ10, and omega-3 fatty acids** complement DMSO's ability to reduce chronic inflammation.

- **Use a Holistic Approach** – Pairing **DMSO with dietary adjustments** (reducing processed foods and increasing anti-inflammatory nutrients) enhances long-term symptom management.

Expected Results

- **First Week** – Reduction in stiffness, improved mobility, and mild pain relief.

- **One to Three Months** – Significant reduction in inflammation, better energy levels, and improved daily function.

- **Long-Term** – Decreased dependency on medications, more stable symptom control, and enhanced quality of life.

DMSO provides **a sustainable alternative to pharmaceuticals,** offering **real relief for chronic inflammatory conditions**. In the next section, we will explore how DMSO can be used for **swelling and bruising, with targeted techniques for rapid reduction.**

8.2.3 Swelling and Bruising: Best Techniques for Rapid Reduction

Swelling and bruising are common symptoms of **injuries, post-surgical recovery, and inflammatory conditions**. While the body naturally resolves these issues over time, excessive swelling can **restrict movement, delay healing, and prolong pain**. Conventional treatments often rely on **NSAIDs, ice therapy, and compression**, which can provide temporary relief but do not address the underlying inflammation at a cellular level. **DMSO offers a more effective solution by directly reducing swelling, improving circulation, and accelerating tissue recovery.**

How DMSO Reduces Swelling and Bruising

DMSO is uniquely effective because of its **ability to penetrate deeply into tissues** and target the root causes of swelling and bruising. It works by:

- **Preventing fluid buildup** – DMSO reduces **capillary permeability**, which helps prevent excess fluid accumulation in injured areas.

- **Enhancing circulation** – By improving microvascular blood flow, DMSO helps **disperse pooled blood and lymphatic congestion**, which accelerates bruise resolution.

- **Breaking down fibrin deposits** – Fibrin is a protein involved in clotting and scar formation. Excess fibrin can contribute to **prolonged swelling and stiffness**. DMSO dissolves fibrin buildup, promoting faster healing.

Recommended DMSO Concentration for Swelling and Bruising

For **general swelling and bruising**, a **50% DMSO solution** (1 part DMSO, 1 part distilled water) is effective. In cases of **severe swelling or hematomas**, a **70% solution** may be used if well tolerated.

Application Protocol for Reducing Swelling and Bruising

1. **Clean the Affected Area**

   o Wash the skin with **mild soap and warm water** to remove contaminants.

   o Ensure the skin is **completely dry** before application.

2. **Apply DMSO to the Swollen or Bruised Area**

   o Using a sterile cotton pad or gauze, **apply a thin layer of DMSO directly over the affected area**.

   o Allow natural absorption—do not rub or massage aggressively.

3. **Let It Absorb and Remove Residue**

   o Leave the solution on for **20 to 30 minutes**, then rinse the area with clean water.

o Avoid covering the treated area with tight clothing or synthetic materials immediately after application.

4. **Repeat as Needed**

    o **For mild swelling or small bruises** → Apply **once daily** until improvement is seen.

    o **For more severe cases** → Apply **twice daily** (morning and evening) for faster results.

Best Practices for Accelerated Recovery

- **Use Cold Therapy in the First 24-48 Hours** – If swelling is due to an acute injury, combining DMSO with ice packs can **prevent excessive fluid buildup**.

- **Elevate the Affected Area** – Keeping the swollen area elevated reduces fluid accumulation and enhances DMSO's effectiveness.

- **Apply After Physical Activity** – If swelling is related to exercise or overuse, using DMSO post-activity can **reduce inflammation before it becomes severe**.

Expected Results

- **First 24 Hours** – Reduction in fluid retention and a decrease in visible bruising.

- **2 to 5 Days** – Significant improvement in swelling, increased comfort, and better range of motion.

- **1 to 2 Weeks** – Near-complete resolution of bruising, minimal residual swelling, and improved tissue function.

DMSO provides **a safe and highly effective approach to managing swelling and bruising,** working **faster and deeper than traditional remedies.** In the next chapter, we will explore how DMSO can be used for **skin and wound care, including protocols for burns, scars, and tissue regeneration.**

Chapter 9:
Skin and Wound Care with DMSO

9.1 USING DMSO FOR SKIN HEALING AND REGENERATION

The skin is the body's **largest organ** and serves as a protective barrier against environmental damage, infections, and physical injuries. However, when the skin is compromised — whether due to **burns, cuts, wounds, or chronic conditions** — healing can be slow and sometimes incomplete, leading to scarring, sensitivity, or long-term damage. **DMSO offers a unique, science-backed approach to skin healing by accelerating tissue regeneration, reducing inflammation, and improving cellular hydration.**

How DMSO Promotes Skin Repair

DMSO is particularly effective for skin healing due to its **exceptional penetration ability** and **anti-inflammatory properties**. Unlike standard topical treatments that act only on the surface, **DMSO absorbs deeply into skin layers, targeting damaged tissues at a cellular level.**

It promotes healing through several mechanisms:

- **Enhancing Cell Regeneration** – DMSO **stimulates fibroblast activity**, which plays a crucial role in collagen production and skin repair. This helps wounds heal faster and minimizes scar formation.

- **Reducing Inflammation and Infection Risk** – DMSO's **natural antimicrobial properties** make it effective against bacteria and fungi, reducing the likelihood of secondary infections.

- **Improving Circulation and Oxygen Delivery** – By increasing blood flow to damaged areas, DMSO ensures that essential nutrients and oxygen reach the skin, **speeding up the healing process**.

- **Minimizing Pain and Skin Irritation** – DMSO has mild anesthetic properties, **soothing discomfort** associated with burns, wounds, and inflammatory skin conditions.

Why DMSO is Different from Conventional Skin Treatments

Most topical skin treatments rely on **moisturizers, steroids, or antibiotics**, which may only provide **temporary relief**. DMSO, on the other hand, **works from within**, addressing the underlying causes of delayed skin healing rather than just masking symptoms.

- Unlike steroid creams, DMSO does not thin the skin over time.

- Unlike antibiotics, DMSO does not contribute to bacterial resistance.

- Unlike traditional moisturizers, DMSO actually improves hydration at a cellular level rather than just sealing in surface moisture.

Safe Application for Skin Healing

Because DMSO **rapidly penetrates the skin**, it must be used **with care** to avoid absorbing unwanted substances. Always ensure:

- The application area is **clean and free of lotions, perfumes, or other chemicals**.

- A sterile cotton pad or gauze is used for application, **never bare hands**.

- The DMSO concentration is **appropriate for the severity of the skin condition** (details provided in targeted protocols in the next sections).

DMSO's ability to **accelerate skin regeneration, prevent infections, and reduce scarring** makes it an **essential tool for wound healing and skin repair**. In the next section, we will explore **specific DMSO protocols for treating burns, cuts, and wound recovery**.

9.2 TARGETED SKIN PROTOCOLS

9.2.1 Burns, Cuts, and Wound Recovery

Skin injuries such as **burns, cuts, and open wounds** can be painful, slow to heal, and prone to infection. While traditional treatments focus on **keeping wounds clean and hydrated**, many fail to address the underlying inflammation, pain, and tissue regeneration needed for complete healing. **DMSO offers a unique, science-backed approach by reducing inflammation, accelerating tissue repair, and enhancing the body's natural healing mechanisms.**

How DMSO Supports Wound Healing

DMSO plays a critical role in **wound recovery** due to its ability to **penetrate deeply into the skin**, targeting damaged tissues at the cellular level. It aids in wound healing by:

- **Reducing Inflammation and Pain** – DMSO blocks inflammatory mediators, helping to control swelling and discomfort while promoting faster healing.

- **Preventing Infection** – With its natural antimicrobial properties, DMSO helps protect wounds from bacterial and fungal infections, reducing the risk of complications.

- **Enhancing Tissue Regeneration** – By stimulating fibroblast activity, DMSO promotes the production of **new collagen and skin cells**, leading to **faster and more complete wound healing**.

- **Minimizing Scarring** – DMSO helps regulate excessive scar tissue formation by balancing collagen synthesis, preventing raised or hardened scars.

Recommended DMSO Concentration for Burns, Cuts, and Wounds

- **For minor cuts, abrasions, and first-degree burns** → Use a **30-50% DMSO solution** (3-5 parts DMSO, 7-5 parts distilled water).

- **For second-degree burns and deeper wounds** → Use a **25-30% DMSO solution** to reduce irritation while still providing therapeutic benefits.

- **For third-degree burns or large open wounds** → Do not apply DMSO directly on raw, exposed tissue. Instead, apply around the wound site to help reduce inflammation in surrounding tissues.

Application Protocol for Burns, Cuts, and Wounds

1. **Clean the Wound Area**
   - Wash the injured area with **mild soap and warm water** to remove any debris or bacteria.

    o Pat dry gently with a clean, sterile cloth.

2. **Apply a Diluted DMSO Solution**

    o Using **a sterile gauze pad or cotton pad**, apply a thin layer of the **appropriate DMSO concentration** over and around the affected area.

    o **Do not rub** — allow the DMSO to be absorbed naturally.

3. **Let the Solution Absorb**

    o Leave the DMSO on for **20 to 30 minutes**, then gently rinse with clean water.

    o If treating a burn, **do not cover the area immediately**; allow the skin to breathe.

4. **Repeat as Needed**

    o **For minor cuts and burns** → Apply **once or twice daily** until healed.

    o **For deeper wounds** → Apply **once daily**, monitoring skin response.

Best Practices for Enhanced Healing

- **Combine with Aloe Vera for Cooling Relief** – Aloe vera gel applied **after DMSO absorption** helps soothe burns and further promotes skin hydration.

- **Support Collagen Formation with Vitamin C** – Since collagen is essential for wound healing, consider supplementing with **vitamin C or applying a vitamin C serum**.

- **Avoid Synthetic Bandages Immediately After Application** – Allow the wound to breathe before covering it with sterile dressings.

Expected Results

- **First 24-48 Hours** – Reduced pain, inflammation, and early signs of healing.

- **3 to 7 Days** – Noticeable skin regeneration, decreased redness, and improved tissue recovery.

- **2 to 4 Weeks** – Complete healing of minor wounds, significant improvement in deeper injuries.

DMSO is a **highly effective tool for accelerating wound recovery, reducing inflammation, and preventing infection**. In the next section, we will explore how **DMSO can be used for scar reduction and skin repair to promote long-term healing.**

9.2.2 Scar Reduction and Skin Repair

Scars form as part of the body's natural healing process, but excessive scarring can lead to **raised, stiff, or discolored skin**, impacting both appearance and mobility. While many conventional treatments focus on **moisturizing or exfoliating the skin**, they often fail to **penetrate deeply enough** to influence tissue remodeling at a cellular level. **DMSO offers a unique solution by softening scar tissue, improving collagen balance, and promoting skin regeneration from within.**

How DMSO Supports Scar Reduction and Skin Repair

DMSO works on scars by **breaking down excess fibrotic tissue**, improving elasticity, and **stimulating the production of healthy skin cells**. Its key benefits include:

- **Softening and Flattening Raised Scars** – DMSO **dissolves hardened collagen fibers**, reducing the appearance of hypertrophic or keloid scars.

- **Regenerating Healthy Skin Cells** – By stimulating **fibroblasts**, DMSO promotes new tissue formation, leading to **smoother, more even skin texture**.

- **Reducing Hyperpigmentation** – DMSO **enhances circulation** to the scarred area, helping to even out skin tone and **fade discoloration** over time.

- **Improving Skin Elasticity** – Unlike some treatments that dry out the skin, DMSO **hydrates and restores** flexibility to scar tissue, making it less rigid.

Recommended DMSO Concentration for Scar Treatment

- **For new scars (less than 6 months old)** → A **50% DMSO solution** (1 part DMSO, 1 part distilled water) is effective for early intervention.

- **For older, more stubborn scars** → A **70% DMSO solution** may be used, but should be introduced gradually to assess skin sensitivity.

- **For sensitive skin areas (face, neck, or thin-skinned regions)** → Start with a **30-50% solution** to minimize irritation.

Application Protocol for Scar Reduction

1. **Prepare the Skin**
   - Wash the affected area with **mild soap and warm water** to remove impurities.
   - Pat the skin completely dry before application.

2. **Apply a Thin Layer of DMSO**
   - Using a **sterile cotton pad or gauze**, apply a thin layer of DMSO directly to the scar.
   - Allow the solution to **absorb naturally** – do not rub aggressively.

3. **Let It Absorb and Rinse If Needed**
    o Leave the solution on for **20 to 30 minutes**, then rinse the area with clean water.
    o If irritation occurs, **reduce concentration or mix DMSO with aloe vera gel**.

4. **Repeat as Needed**
    o **For new scars** → Apply **once daily for 4 to 6 weeks**.
    o **For older scars** → Apply **twice daily (morning and evening)** for a minimum of **8 to 12 weeks**.

Best Practices for Optimal Scar Healing

- **Pair with Vitamin E or Rosehip Oil** – After DMSO absorption, apply **vitamin E oil or rosehip seed oil** to nourish and support skin repair.

- **Massage Gently for Improved Circulation** – Light circular massage around the scar (after DMSO has been absorbed) can **enhance collagen remodeling**.

- **Avoid Sun Exposure** – Healing skin is sensitive to UV damage; **use sun protection** to prevent further discoloration.

Expected Results

- **First 2-4 Weeks** – Softening of scar tissue, improved skin texture, and less noticeable discoloration.

- **4-8 Weeks** – Flattening of raised scars, more even skin tone, and improved elasticity.

- **8-12 Weeks** – Significant reduction in scar appearance, increased skin smoothness, and overall tissue repair.

DMSO provides a **non-invasive yet highly effective approach** to reducing scars and improving skin quality. In the next section, we will explore **how to manage skin sensitivity and avoid irritation when using DMSO for topical applications.**

9.2.3 Managing Sensitivity and Avoiding Irritation

While **DMSO is a powerful tool for skin healing,** its ability to penetrate deeply into tissues means it must be used carefully to avoid irritation. Some individuals experience **redness, dryness, or mild itching,** especially when first introducing DMSO into their routine. These effects are usually temporary and manageable with the right precautions. Understanding how to **apply DMSO correctly, choose the right concentration, and minimize irritation** can ensure safe and effective use.

Why Skin Sensitivity Occurs with DMSO

DMSO interacts directly with skin cells and can **enhance the absorption of environmental contaminants, lotions, or chemical residues.** Sensitivity can arise due to:

- **Overly High Concentrations** – Stronger solutions (above **70% DMSO**) may cause **dryness, redness, or a mild burning sensation,** particularly in sensitive individuals.

- **Impurities Absorbed Through the Skin** – If applied over unclean skin or with contaminated materials, DMSO can transport harmful substances directly into the body.

- **Prolonged Contact** – Leaving DMSO on the skin for extended periods (beyond **30 minutes**) may increase irritation in some cases.

- **Natural Individual Sensitivity** – Some people's skin is simply more reactive, especially in delicate areas such as the **face, neck, or inner arms**.

How to Minimize Skin Irritation

1. **Use the Right Concentration**

   o **For sensitive skin areas (face, neck, inner arms, or thin-skinned regions)** → Start with a **30% to 50% DMSO solution**.

   o **For general skin application** → A **50% solution** is well tolerated by most individuals.

   o **For tougher areas (knees, elbows, or scars on thicker skin)** → A **70% solution** may be used but should be introduced gradually.

2. **Always Apply to Clean, Dry Skin**

   o Wash the area with **mild soap and warm water** before applying DMSO.

   o Avoid **chemical-laden lotions, perfumes, or synthetic fabrics** on the application site, as DMSO can carry their components into the bloodstream.

3. **Limit Contact Time**

- o Let the solution absorb for **20 to 30 minutes** before rinsing off with **clean water**.
- o Avoid leaving DMSO on overnight unless specifically directed for a therapeutic application.

4. **Moisturize After Application**

- o If dryness or irritation occurs, apply **a natural moisturizer** such as **aloe vera gel, vitamin E oil, or jojoba oil** after the DMSO has fully absorbed.
- o **Avoid conventional creams or lotions**, as they often contain synthetic chemicals that DMSO may transport into the skin.

5. **Test on a Small Area First**

- o Before using DMSO on large areas, apply a small amount to a **patch of skin** (such as the inner forearm) and monitor for **24 hours**.
- o If irritation occurs, dilute further before applying again.

6. **Rotate Application Sites**

- o If using DMSO **daily**, consider rotating application areas to **give the skin time to recover**.
- o For long-term use, **take a break** (such as 1-2 weeks off after 6-8 weeks of continuous use) to prevent sensitivity buildup.

What to Do If Irritation Occurs

- **Mild redness or tingling** → Reduce concentration and apply a **soothing agent** like aloe vera or chamomile extract.
- **Persistent dryness or peeling** → Apply **a few drops of coconut oil or vitamin E** after DMSO absorption.
- **Severe irritation or allergic reaction** → Discontinue use and consult a healthcare professional.

Expected Results with Proper Use

- **First Applications** – Mild warmth or tingling is normal and usually subsides within a few minutes.
- **One to Two Weeks** – Skin adapts to DMSO use, with reduced sensitivity and improved healing benefits.
- **Long-Term** – Minimal irritation with continued proper use, healthier skin regeneration, and enhanced therapeutic effects.

Chapter 10:
DMSO for Respiratory and Immune Health

10.1: SUPPORTING RESPIRATORY HEALTH

Expanding on the use of **DMSO** for respiratory health, it's important to consider the incorporation of **natural remedies** that have been traditionally used for their respiratory benefits. For instance, **thyme** has been recognized for its expectorant properties, helping to clear mucus from the airways, while **licorice root** is known for its soothing effect on irritated throat and bronchial tubes. When these are combined with DMSO, their bioavailability and efficacy can be significantly enhanced, offering a potent natural solution for respiratory discomforts.

It's crucial to use only pharmaceutical-grade DMSO and organic herbs to ensure purity and safety. Additionally, always conduct a patch test with DMSO on a small skin area before proceeding with these treatments, especially if you have sensitive skin or are prone to allergies. The synergy between DMSO and these natural remedies offers a powerful approach to managing respiratory health, but it's essential to listen to your body and consult with a healthcare professional if symptoms persist or worsen. These protocols are designed to support and complement traditional medical treatments, not replace them. By leveraging the unique properties of DMSO in combination with time-honored natural remedies, you can create a holistic regimen that supports respiratory health and enhances your body's natural healing capabilities.

10.1.1: Recipes for Respiratory Health

DMSO and Thyme Steam Inhalation

Objective: To create a steam inhalation blend using DMSO and thyme essential oil, aimed at supporting respiratory health by leveraging thyme's natural expectorant and antibacterial properties, enhanced with the deep tissue penetration of DMSO.

Beneficial Effects: This steam inhalation is designed to help clear nasal passages, ease breathing, and provide relief from respiratory conditions such as colds, coughs, and sinusitis. Thyme's antimicrobial properties help fight respiratory infections, while DMSO enhances the delivery of thyme's therapeutic compounds into the respiratory system.

Ingredients:

- 1 teaspoon of 99.9% pure DMSO

- 3-5 drops of thyme essential oil

- 1 bowl of boiling water (approximately 2 quarts)

Portions: This recipe is for a single steam inhalation session.

Step-by-Step Instructions:

1. Boil 2 quarts of water and carefully pour it into a large, heat-resistant bowl. Allow the water to cool slightly, just enough so that steam is still rising but not so hot as to pose a risk of scalding.

2. Add 1 teaspoon of 99.9% pure DMSO to the hot water. Stir gently with a heat-resistant spoon or stirrer to ensure the DMSO is well distributed throughout the water.

3. Add 3-5 drops of thyme essential oil to the mixture. Stir again gently to disperse the essential oil in the water.

4. Position yourself comfortably in front of the bowl, at a safe distance to avoid any risk of steam burns.

5. Drape a large towel over your head and the bowl, creating a tent that traps the steam.

6. Close your eyes and lean over the bowl, inhaling the steam deeply through your nose for about 5-10 minutes. Adjust your distance from the bowl as needed to regulate the intensity of the steam inhalation.

7. Pause and take breaks if needed, especially if the steam feels too intense or if you need to catch your breath.

Application Mode:

- Use this steam inhalation once daily, preferably in the evening before bedtime, to help alleviate respiratory discomfort and promote restful sleep.

- For acute conditions, the steam inhalation can be used up to twice daily, reducing to once daily as symptoms improve.

Precautions:

- Ensure the water is not too hot before adding DMSO and thyme essential oil to prevent degradation of their therapeutic properties.

- Always conduct a patch test with diluted DMSO on your skin before using it in the inhalation to check for any adverse reactions.

- Thyme essential oil is potent; start with fewer drops to test for sensitivity before increasing to the recommended amount.

- Avoid direct contact of the hot water and steam with your skin to prevent burns.

- Individuals with asthma or other respiratory conditions should consult with a healthcare professional before using steam inhalation therapy.

Additional Tips:

- Keep the room free from drafts to maximize the benefits of the steam inhalation.

- Hydrate well before and after the steam inhalation to help thin mucus and support the body's natural respiratory functions.

- Consider incorporating other supportive practices such as staying well-hydrated, using a humidifier in dry environments, and practicing gentle breathing exercises to enhance respiratory health.

DMSO and Licorice Root Syrup

Objective: To create a therapeutic syrup combining DMSO and licorice root, designed to support respiratory health by leveraging the anti-inflammatory and soothing properties of licorice root enhanced with the deep tissue penetration of DMSO.

Beneficial Effects: This syrup aims to soothe irritated throats, reduce coughing, and support overall respiratory health through the combined action of licorice root, known for its expectorant and soothing properties, and DMSO, which enhances the delivery of licorice's beneficial compounds.

Ingredients:

- 1/4 cup of dried licorice root

- 2 cups of water

- 1 tablespoon of 99.9% pure DMSO

- 1/2 cup of honey (to sweeten and provide additional antimicrobial benefits)

Portions: Yields approximately 2 cups of syrup.

Step-by-Step Instructions:

1. Combine 2 cups of water and 1/4 cup of dried licorice root in a medium saucepan. Bring the mixture to a boil over high heat.

2. Once boiling, reduce the heat to low and let the mixture simmer uncovered for 30 minutes, allowing the water to reduce by half and the licorice root to infuse thoroughly.

3. After simmering, remove the saucepan from the heat and strain the mixture using a fine mesh strainer or cheesecloth, discarding the licorice root solids. Allow the liquid to cool to room temperature.

4. When the licorice infusion has cooled, stir in 1 tablespoon of 99.9% pure DMSO. Mix thoroughly to ensure the DMSO is well integrated.

5. Add 1/2 cup of honey to the mixture and stir until the honey is completely dissolved, providing a sweet flavor and additional soothing properties to the syrup.

6. Transfer the syrup into a clean glass bottle or jar with a tight-fitting lid for storage.

Application Mode:

- Shake the bottle well before each use to ensure the ingredients are well mixed.

- Take 1 tablespoon of the DMSO and Licorice Root Syrup up to three times daily, especially when experiencing throat irritation or coughing.

- The syrup can be taken directly or diluted in a small amount of warm water or tea for a soothing drink.

Precautions:

- Perform a patch test with diluted DMSO on a small area of skin before ingesting the syrup to check for any adverse reactions.

- Consult with a healthcare professional before using this syrup, especially if you are pregnant, nursing, have high blood pressure, or are on medication, as licorice root can interact with certain medications and conditions.

- Do not exceed the recommended dosage, as excessive consumption of licorice root can lead to adverse effects.

Additional Tips:

- Store the syrup in a cool, dark place, such as a refrigerator, to preserve its potency and freshness. The syrup can be stored for up to 2 weeks.

- If the taste of licorice is too strong, the amount of honey can be adjusted to suit personal preference, or a small amount of lemon juice can be added to balance the flavor.

- For enhanced respiratory support, consider pairing the syrup with other natural remedies such as ginger tea or eucalyptus steam inhalation.

10.2: Enhancing Immune Response with DMSO

In the quest to enhance immune response, the integration of **DMSO** with **natural supplements** emerges as a compelling strategy. This approach is not merely about combining substances but about harnessing the unique properties of DMSO to improve the bioavailability and efficacy of immune-boosting supplements. For instance, when **DMSO** is mixed with **Vitamin C**, it can facilitate deeper penetration of this potent antioxidant into the cells, thereby amplifying its immune-strengthening effects. The preparation of a **DMSO and Vitamin C Serum** involves dissolving high-quality, non-GMO Vitamin C powder in distilled water to create a saturated solution. To this, add pharmaceutical-grade DMSO in a ratio that ensures a final concentration of 25% DMSO. This concoction can be applied topically to the forearm or the soles of the feet, areas with thinner skin for optimal absorption.

Similarly, the combination of **DMSO** with **Magnesium Supplement Gel** offers a dual benefit. Magnesium is crucial for numerous biochemical reactions in the body, including those that support immune function. By creating a gel that combines magnesium oil with DMSO, one can enhance the transdermal uptake of magnesium, thus directly supporting the body's natural defense mechanisms. Start with a base of magnesium oil, available from health stores, and mix it with DMSO at a 1:1 ratio. This gel can be applied to areas of the body with muscle mass, such as the thighs or arms, facilitating not only immune support but also muscle relaxation.

The inclusion of **Zinc Oxide Cream** with DMSO in the regimen taps into zinc's vital role in immune health. Zinc supports the immune system's ability to fight off invading bacteria and viruses. Creating a **Zinc Oxide Cream** involves blending zinc oxide powder with a carrier oil, such as coconut oil, to form a paste. Adding DMSO to this mixture enhances the skin's absorption of zinc. The cream can be applied to the chest or back, providing a localized area for absorption that directly benefits the respiratory system, a primary entry point for pathogens.

It's imperative to use only the highest quality ingredients when creating these mixtures. Opt for pharmaceutical-grade DMSO and certified organic or non-GMO supplements to ensure purity and safety. Moreover, precise measurement is crucial to achieving the desired concentration and efficacy of the final product. Utilizing digital scales for solid ingredients and graduated cylinders for liquids can ensure accuracy.

Before applying any new DMSO mixture, conducting a patch test is essential to gauge individual skin sensitivity. Apply a small amount of the prepared solution to a discreet area and monitor for any adverse reactions over 24 hours. This precautionary step is vital to ensure compatibility and prevent skin irritation.

The frequency of application and the duration of use should be tailored to individual needs and responses. Some may benefit from daily application, while others might find intermittent use sufficient. Observing the body's reaction and adjusting accordingly is key to optimizing the immune-boosting benefits of these DMSO-enhanced supplements.

Engaging with a healthcare professional knowledgeable about DMSO and its use with supplements can provide additional insights and guidance tailored to individual health profiles. This professional oversight ensures that the incorporation of DMSO into an immune support regimen complements existing health protocols and addresses specific needs without interfering with other treatments.

By meticulously combining DMSO with selected supplements, individuals can create a personalized toolkit for immune support. This proactive approach empowers individuals to harness the synergistic potential of DMSO and natural supplements, potentially enhancing their body's resilience against illness and promoting overall well-being.

10.2.1: Immune-Boosting Recipes

DMSO and Elderberry Extract Elixir

Objective: To create a potent elixir using DMSO and elderberry extract aimed at boosting the immune system, particularly beneficial during cold and flu season.

Benefits: This elixir combines the immune-supporting properties of elderberry with the enhanced absorption qualities of DMSO, offering a powerful tool for preventing and fighting off viral infections.

Ingredients:

- 1/4 cup of elderberry extract

- 2 tablespoons of 99.9% pure DMSO

- 1/2 cup of distilled water

- 2 tablespoons of raw honey (optional, for taste)

- Glass bottle for storage

Portions: Yields approximately 1 cup of elixir.

Step-by-Step Instructions:

1. In a clean glass mixing bowl, combine 1/4 cup of elderberry extract with 1/2 cup of distilled water. Stir gently to ensure the elderberry extract is fully dissolved in the water.

2. Slowly add 2 tablespoons of 99.9% pure DMSO to the elderberry and water mixture. Stir continuously for a few minutes to ensure the DMSO is fully integrated. The DMSO will act as a carrier, enhancing the absorption of the elderberry's beneficial compounds.

3. If desired, add 2 tablespoons of raw honey to the mixture. Stir well until the honey is completely dissolved. Honey adds a natural sweetness and offers additional antimicrobial and soothing properties.

4. Carefully pour the final mixture into a glass bottle. Seal the bottle tightly with a lid to prevent any contamination or evaporation.

Application Mode:

- Shake the bottle well before each use to ensure the ingredients are well mixed.

- Take 1 tablespoon of the DMSO and Elderberry Elixir daily during cold and flu season for immune support.

- If experiencing early symptoms of a cold or flu, the dosage can be increased to 1 tablespoon up to 4 times daily.

Precautions:

- Perform a patch test with diluted DMSO on a small area of skin before consuming the elixir to ensure no adverse reaction occurs.

- Consult with a healthcare professional before using this elixir, especially if you are pregnant, nursing, have a medical condition, or are taking any medication, as elderberry and DMSO may interact with certain conditions and medications.

- Do not exceed the recommended dosage without consulting a healthcare provider.

Additional Tips:

- Store the elixir in a cool, dark place, such as a refrigerator, to maintain its potency and freshness. Use within 2 weeks for optimal benefits.

- For children or those with sensitive palates, the elixir can be diluted in a small amount of water or juice to make it more palatable.

- Incorporate other immune-boosting practices into your routine, such as maintaining a healthy diet rich in fruits and vegetables, staying hydrated, and getting adequate sleep, to further support your immune system.

DMSO and Astragalus Root Tonic

Objective: To create a tonic using DMSO and Astragalus Root aimed at boosting the immune system.

Benefits: This tonic leverages the immunomodulating properties of Astragalus Root, known for its ability to enhance the body's resistance to infections. Combined with DMSO, it ensures deeper absorption and efficacy, promoting overall immune health and resilience.

Ingredients:

- 1/4 cup of dried Astragalus Root

- 2 cups of water

- 1 tablespoon of 99.9% pure DMSO

- 1/4 cup of raw honey (optional, for taste)

Portions: Yields approximately 2 cups of tonic.

Step-by-Step Instructions:

1. Place 1/4 cup of dried Astragalus Root into a medium saucepan.

2. Add 2 cups of water to the saucepan, ensuring the Astragalus Root is fully submerged.

3. Bring the water to a boil over high heat, then reduce to a simmer. Cover and let simmer for 1 hour, allowing the Astragalus Root to steep and its properties to infuse into the water.

4. After simmering, remove the saucepan from the heat. Strain the mixture through a fine mesh strainer or cheesecloth into a large glass bowl, discarding the Astragalus Root solids.

5. Allow the strained liquid to cool to room temperature. Once cooled, add 1 tablespoon of 99.9% pure DMSO to the Astragalus infusion. Stir thoroughly to ensure the DMSO is well integrated.

6. If desired, stir in 1/4 cup of raw honey to the mixture to sweeten.

7. Transfer the tonic into a glass bottle or jar with a tight-fitting lid for storage.

Application Mode:

- Shake the bottle well before each use to ensure the ingredients are well mixed.

- Take 1 tablespoon of the DMSO and Astragalus Root Tonic up to two times daily.

- For best results, consume the tonic in the morning and evening.

Precautions:

- Conduct a patch test with diluted DMSO on a small area of skin before ingesting the tonic to check for any adverse reactions.

- Consult with a healthcare professional before using this tonic, especially if you are pregnant, nursing, or have any underlying health conditions.

- Do not exceed the recommended dosage of DMSO.

Additional Tips:

- Store the tonic in a cool, dark place, such as a refrigerator, to preserve its potency and freshness. The tonic can be stored for up to 2 weeks.

- For an additional immune boost, consider incorporating other immune-supporting practices into your routine, such as maintaining a healthy diet, getting regular exercise, and ensuring adequate sleep.

- If the taste of the tonic is too strong, consider diluting it with a small amount of water or herbal tea before consumption.

10.3: DMSO AND NATURAL OILS BENEFITS

Expanding upon the synergy between DMSO and natural oils, it's crucial to delve into the specifics of how these combinations can be optimized for enhanced benefits. The focus here is on creating mixtures that not only maximize therapeutic effects but also ensure safety and ease of application. **Jojoba oil**, renowned for its moisturizing properties, and **avocado oil**, celebrated for its rich antioxidant content, stand out as prime candidates for combination with DMSO. When blending DMSO with these oils, the goal is to achieve a formulation that supports skin health while delivering the deep tissue penetration for which DMSO is known.

When utilizing these DMSO-oil mixtures, several application tips can optimize their effectiveness. Firstly, clean the application area with a gentle, non-alcoholic cleanser to remove any barriers that could impede absorption. Secondly, apply the mixture in a well-ventilated area, as DMSO can produce a garlic-like odor as it metabolizes. Lastly, consider wearing gloves when applying the mixture to avoid transdermal absorption through the fingers, unless treating the hands directly.

Monitoring the skin's response to these treatments is essential. Look for any signs of irritation or discomfort, which may indicate a need to adjust the DMSO concentration. Additionally, because DMSO can enhance the absorption of substances through the skin, ensure that the application area is free from any harmful chemicals or residues.

Incorporating DMSO with jojoba and avocado oils presents a powerful approach to natural healing and skin care. By understanding the properties of each component and following precise mixing and application guidelines, individuals can harness these combinations' full therapeutic potential. Whether seeking to moisturize dry skin, reduce inflammation, or enhance the delivery of beneficial compounds, these DMSO-oil mixtures offer a versatile and effective solution. Always remember, the key to successful application lies in careful preparation, mindful application, and attentive observation of the body's response.

10.3.1: Recipes with Natural Oils

DMSO and Jojoba Oil Serum

Objective: To create a nourishing serum that combines the deep tissue penetration abilities of DMSO with the moisturizing and healing properties of jojoba oil, aimed at enhancing skin health and appearance.

Benefits: This serum harnesses the moisturizing power of jojoba oil, which closely mimics the skin's natural oils, along with the enhanced absorption properties of DMSO. It's designed to deeply nourish the skin, reduce the appearance of fine lines and wrinkles, and improve overall skin texture.

Ingredients:

- 2 tablespoons of 99.9% pure DMSO

- 1/4 cup of cold-pressed jojoba oil

- 5 drops of lavender essential oil (optional, for scent and additional skin benefits)

- Dark glass dropper bottle for storage

Portions: Yields approximately 4 ounces of serum.

Step-by-Step Instructions:

1. In a clean, dry glass bowl, combine 1/4 cup of cold-pressed jojoba oil with 5 drops of lavender essential oil (if using). Use a glass stirrer to gently mix the oils together, ensuring the lavender oil is evenly distributed throughout the jojoba oil.

2. Slowly add 2 tablespoons of 99.9% pure DMSO to the oil mixture. Stir continuously for a few minutes to ensure that the DMSO is fully integrated with the jojoba and lavender oils. The mixture should appear homogeneous and smooth.

3. Using a small funnel, carefully transfer the serum into a dark glass dropper bottle. The dark glass helps to preserve the integrity of the oils and DMSO by protecting them from light degradation.

4. Seal the dropper bottle tightly with its lid to prevent any air exposure, which could compromise the serum's effectiveness.

Application Mode:

- Cleanse your face thoroughly and pat dry before application.

- Shake the dropper bottle gently before each use to ensure the ingredients are well mixed.

- Apply 3-5 drops of the DMSO and Jojoba Oil Serum to your fingertips and gently massage into the face and neck, focusing on areas with fine lines, wrinkles, or dry patches.

- Use the serum twice daily, in the morning and evening, for best results.

Precautions:

- Conduct a patch test on a small, inconspicuous area of skin 24 hours before applying broadly to ensure no adverse reaction occurs.

- Avoid direct contact with eyes, mucous membranes, and open wounds.

- Use the serum in a well-ventilated area to minimize inhalation of DMSO fumes.

- If pregnant, nursing, or suffering from any medical condition, consult a healthcare professional before use.

Additional Tips:

- Store the serum in a cool, dark place to maintain its potency. A refrigerator can extend its shelf life but is not necessary.

- If your skin feels oily after application, gently blot the excess with a clean tissue.

- For an added boost of hydration, consider applying the serum while your skin is still slightly damp from cleansing.

- Complement the use of this serum with a daily SPF to protect the skin from further damage and support the healing process.

DMSO and Avocado Oil Cream

Objective: Craft a nourishing cream combining the deep tissue penetration of DMSO with the hydrating and healing properties of avocado oil, aimed at enhancing skin health and providing relief from dryness and irritation.

Benefits: This cream harnesses the hydrating power of avocado oil, rich in vitamins A, D, and E, known for their skin-soothing and healing properties. When combined with DMSO, it facilitates deeper absorption of these nutrients, promoting enhanced skin repair, hydration, and elasticity.

Ingredients:

- 2 tablespoons of 99.9% pure DMSO

- 1/2 cup of avocado oil

- 1/4 cup of coconut oil (as a solid base)

- 2 tablespoons of beeswax (to thicken the cream)

- 10 drops of lavender essential oil (for additional skin healing benefits)

- Glass mixing bowl

- Glass or metal storage container with a lid

Portions: Yields approximately 8 ounces of cream.

Step-by-Step Instructions:

1. In a small saucepan, bring water to a simmer. Place a glass mixing bowl over the saucepan to create a double boiler.

2. Add the coconut oil and beeswax to the glass mixing bowl. Stir occasionally with a wooden or glass stirrer until completely melted and combined.

3. Remove the glass mixing bowl from the heat and let it cool for 2-3 minutes, ensuring it's not too hot before proceeding to the next step to preserve the therapeutic qualities of the DMSO and avocado oil.

4. Slowly add 2 tablespoons of DMSO to the melted oil and beeswax mixture, stirring constantly to ensure a homogeneous blend.

5. Add 1/2 cup of avocado oil to the mixture. Continue stirring to ensure the avocado oil is evenly distributed throughout the cream.

6. Add 10 drops of lavender essential oil to the mixture for additional skin healing benefits and a pleasant scent. Stir well.

7. Carefully pour the mixture into a glass or metal storage container. Allow it to cool and solidify at room temperature, away from direct sunlight.

8. Once cooled and solidified, seal the container with a lid to prevent contamination and degradation of the cream.

Application Mode:

- Clean and dry the area of skin where the cream will be applied.

- Using clean fingers or a spatula, apply a small amount of the DMSO and Avocado Oil Cream to the skin.

- Gently massage the cream into the skin in a circular motion until it is absorbed.

- Apply the cream twice daily, in the morning and evening, for best results.

Precautions:

- Conduct a patch test on a small area to check for any allergic reactions.

- Avoid using near eyes, mucous membranes, or on open wounds.

- Use in a well-ventilated area and avoid inhaling the fumes directly.

- Consult with a healthcare professional before using, especially if pregnant, nursing, or have a medical condition.

Additional Tips:

- Store the cream in a cool, dark place to maintain its potency over time.

- If the cream hardens too much, gently warm the container in a bowl of warm water before use.

- For enhanced skin benefits, ensure a consistent skincare routine and consider pairing the cream with a gentle cleanser and sunscreen during the day.

Chapter 11:
Integrative DMSO Protocols

In the realm of natural healing, the integration of DMSO with other therapies presents a promising frontier for enhancing therapeutic outcomes. This approach leverages the unique properties of DMSO to augment the efficacy of supplements, herbal remedies, and essential oils, thereby creating a synergistic effect that can significantly improve health outcomes. When considering the use of DMSO in conjunction with supplements such as Vitamin C, Magnesium, or Zinc, it is crucial to understand the biochemical interactions that may occur. For instance, DMSO's ability to penetrate cellular membranes can increase the cellular uptake of Vitamin C, a potent antioxidant, thereby enhancing its immune-boosting and reparative functions. Similarly, when DMSO is combined with Magnesium, the transdermal delivery of this essential mineral can be optimized, potentially improving outcomes in conditions related to Magnesium deficiency such as muscle cramps and fatigue.

The application of DMSO with herbal remedies and essential oils also opens up avenues for targeted therapeutic effects. For example, combining DMSO with Sage Oil Infusion can amplify the anti-inflammatory and antioxidant properties of sage, making it a potent remedy for inflammatory conditions and oxidative stress. Meanwhile, a DMSO and Fennel Seed Gel blend could offer relief in digestive discomforts, leveraging DMSO's transdermal delivery to enhance the antispasmodic effects of fennel. It is important to note that while DMSO can enhance the penetration and efficacy of these compounds, careful consideration must be given to the concentration of DMSO used, as well as the purity and quality of the combined substances to avoid skin irritation or adverse reactions.

Moreover, the complementary use of DMSO with over-the-counter pain relievers like White Willow Bark Extract, which contains salicin — a precursor to salicylic acid, can offer a natural alternative to synthetic pain medications with fewer side effects. This combination can be particularly beneficial for managing mild to moderate pain while also reducing inflammation through a more natural pathway.

In crafting these integrative protocols, it is essential to start with a thorough understanding of the individual's health status, potential allergies, and specific health goals. Personalization of these protocols allows for a more targeted approach, maximizing the benefits while minimizing risks. The preparation of these blends, whether it be a serum, gel, or cream, requires meticulous attention to detail to ensure that the final product is both safe and effective. For instance, when creating a DMSO and Vitamin C Serum, the correct ratio of DMSO to Vitamin C must be calculated to ensure stability and efficacy of the serum over time. Similarly, when preparing a DMSO and Magnesium Supplement Gel, the consistency and pH of the gel should be adjusted to ensure optimal skin compatibility and magnesium absorption.

The exploration of DMSO's integrative use with other therapies is not without challenges. The variability in individual responses to DMSO and combined therapies necessitates a cautious and informed approach. Continuous monitoring and adjustment of the protocols may be required to achieve the desired therapeutic outcomes. Additionally, the importance of consulting healthcare professionals before embarking on any new treatment regimen cannot be overstated. This ensures that the integrative use of DMSO aligns with the individual's overall health plan and avoids potential contraindications with existing medications or conditions.

The meticulous selection of ingredients for each blend is paramount. For instance, when combining DMSO with essential oils such as Lavender or Peppermint for a calming or cooling effect, respectively, the ratio of DMSO to essential oil must be carefully calibrated to prevent skin irritation while ensuring therapeutic efficacy. This balance is crucial, as too high a concentration of essential oils can lead to adverse reactions, whereas too low may render the mixture ineffective. Furthermore, the method of application plays a significant role in the effectiveness of the treatment. Techniques such as gentle massage, compress application, or direct topical application can influence how well the active ingredients are absorbed and, consequently, their therapeutic impact.

In addition to the physical preparation of these blends, the timing and frequency of application are critical factors that can significantly affect outcomes. For conditions such as chronic inflammation or pain, a regular application schedule may be necessary to maintain therapeutic levels of the active compounds in the body. Conversely, for acute conditions, such as a sudden onset of muscle soreness or a headache, a single, more concentrated application may be sufficient to provide relief.

The integration of DMSO with supplements and natural remedies also underscores the importance of quality assurance in the sourcing of all components. Ensuring that the DMSO is of pharmaceutical grade and that herbs and essential oils are organic and free from contaminants is essential for safety and efficacy. This attention to quality not only enhances the therapeutic value of the final product but also minimizes the risk of contamination or adverse reactions.

Education on the proper storage and handling of DMSO and the final blends is another critical aspect. DMSO is a potent solvent that can dissolve certain types of plastic, which means that storage in glass containers is preferable to maintain the integrity of the solution. Similarly, the final blends should be stored in amber or opaque containers to protect them from light degradation, particularly if essential oils are part of the formulation.

Finally, the journey of integrating DMSO with other therapies is one of continuous learning and adaptation. As new research emerges and as individuals share their experiences, the protocols may evolve to incorporate new insights or to better address the needs of those seeking natural healing solutions. Engaging with a community of practitioners and individuals who are exploring the use of DMSO in integrative protocols can provide valuable support and insights. This collaborative approach not only enriches the individual's healing journey but also contributes to the broader understanding of how DMSO can be used safely and effectively as part of an integrative approach to health and wellness.

11.1: DMSO WITH SUPPLEMENTS

When considering the integration of DMSO with dietary supplements such as **Vitamin C** and **Magnesium**, it's essential to approach with a methodical and informed strategy to maximize benefits and minimize any potential risks. The unique property of DMSO to enhance cellular absorption can be leveraged to improve the bioavailability of these supplements, potentially leading to more pronounced health benefits. For instance, when combining DMSO with **Vitamin C**, a powerful antioxidant known for its immune-boosting and skin health properties, the mixture could be prepared by dissolving a specific amount of Vitamin C powder in a solution of DMSO and distilled water. The ideal ratio might be 1 part Vitamin C to 3 parts DMSO, adjusted according to individual tolerance and health objectives. This concoction could then be applied topically to areas of the skin where absorption is optimal, such as the inner wrists or forearms, ensuring that the skin is clean and free from any barriers that might impede absorption.

Similarly, when integrating **Magnesium**—an essential mineral involved in over 300 biochemical reactions in the body, including muscle and nerve function, blood glucose control, and blood pressure regulation—with DMSO, the goal is to create a transdermal application that bypasses gastrointestinal routes, potentially reducing digestive disturbances and enhancing uptake. A practical approach might involve mixing Magnesium oil, which is Magnesium chloride dissolved in water, with DMSO at a ratio that ensures skin safety and maximizes absorption. A starting point could be a mixture of 70% Magnesium oil to 30% DMSO, applied to large areas of the body such as the legs or arms, where it can be easily absorbed without causing irritation.

For those looking to support bone health, a blend of DMSO with **Vitamin D3** and **Calcium** supplements could be considered. Vitamin D3 enhances Calcium absorption in the gut, but when mixed with DMSO, the transdermal route could be an innovative approach to support bone density. This would involve dissolving Vitamin D3 and Calcium in a DMSO solution, carefully calculating the dosage to avoid exceeding recommended daily allowances, and applying the mixture to the skin, ideally in areas where bone health support is desired, such as the lower back or hips.

Incorporating **Zinc**, an essential mineral known for its role in immune function, wound healing, and DNA synthesis, into a DMSO protocol involves careful consideration of Zinc's various forms and their solubility in DMSO. A Zinc sulfate solution mixed with DMSO could be applied to the skin to potentially support immune health and skin integrity, especially during times of increased need such as cold and flu season or in the healing of wounds.

The application technique is crucial for all these protocols. The skin must be clean and dry before application, and the use of gloves is recommended when handling DMSO to prevent unwanted substances from being carried through the skin. Applying these mixtures should be done gently, using a soft brush or a glass dropper to avoid direct contact with plastics, which DMSO can dissolve. After application, allowing the skin to air dry naturally will enable the DMSO and supplement mixture to penetrate effectively.

It's imperative to start with lower concentrations of DMSO when first integrating it with supplements to assess tolerance and gradually increase as deemed suitable based on personal health objectives and responses. Regular consultation with a healthcare provider is advisable to monitor health status and adjust protocols as necessary. Additionally, keeping a detailed journal of formulations, dosages, and responses can be invaluable in fine-tuning the approach for optimal health outcomes.

11.1.1: DMSO Supplement Recipes

DMSO and Vitamin C Serum

Objective: To create a serum that combines the antioxidant power of Vitamin C with the deep tissue penetration of DMSO, aimed at enhancing skin health by promoting collagen production and reducing signs of aging.

Benefits: This serum leverages the collagen-boosting and antioxidant properties of Vitamin C, along with the enhanced absorption qualities of DMSO, to improve skin texture, reduce the appearance of fine lines and wrinkles, and protect against environmental damage.

Ingredients:

- 1 tablespoon of Vitamin C powder (L-ascorbic acid)

- 1/4 cup of distilled water

- 1 teaspoon of 99.9% pure DMSO

- 1 tablespoon of glycerin (to add moisture)

- Dark glass dropper bottle for storage

Portions: Yields approximately 4 ounces of serum.

Step-by-Step Instructions:

1. In a clean, dry glass bowl, dissolve 1 tablespoon of Vitamin C powder in 1/4 cup of distilled water. Stir gently with a glass stirrer until the Vitamin C powder is fully dissolved.

2. Add 1 teaspoon of 99.9% pure DMSO to the Vitamin C solution. Stir thoroughly for a few minutes to ensure the DMSO is fully integrated. DMSO will enhance the penetration of Vitamin C into the skin.

3. Mix in 1 tablespoon of glycerin to the solution. Stir until the glycerin is completely blended. Glycerin will help to add moisture to the skin, making the serum more hydrating.

4. Using a small funnel, carefully transfer the serum into a dark glass dropper bottle. The dark glass helps to protect the Vitamin C from light, which can degrade its potency.

5. Seal the dropper bottle tightly with its lid to prevent any air exposure, which could compromise the serum's effectiveness.

Application Mode:

- Cleanse your face thoroughly and pat dry before application.

- Shake the dropper bottle gently before each use to ensure the ingredients are well mixed.

- Apply 3-5 drops of the DMSO and Vitamin C Serum to your fingertips and gently massage into the face and neck, focusing on areas with fine lines, wrinkles, or uneven skin tone.

- Use the serum once daily, preferably in the evening, as Vitamin C can make the skin more sensitive to sunlight.

Precautions:

- Conduct a patch test on a small, inconspicuous area of skin 24 hours before applying broadly to ensure no adverse reaction occurs.

- Avoid direct contact with eyes, mucous membranes, and open wounds.

- Use the serum in a well-ventilated area to minimize inhalation of DMSO fumes.

- If pregnant, nursing, or suffering from any medical condition, consult a healthcare professional before use.

Additional Tips:

- Store the serum in a cool, dark place to maintain its potency. Refrigeration can extend its shelf life but is not necessary.

- If the serum causes any irritation or discomfort, reduce the frequency of application or discontinue use and consult a healthcare professional.

- For enhanced skin protection, complement the use of this serum with a daily SPF moisturizer during the day.

DMSO and Magnesium Supplement Gel

Objective: To create a magnesium supplement gel that utilizes DMSO for enhanced skin absorption, aimed at providing relief from muscle soreness and improving overall magnesium levels in the body.

Benefits: This gel combines the muscle-relaxing and magnesium-boosting benefits of magnesium with the deep penetration capabilities of DMSO, offering a natural solution for muscle soreness, cramps, and improving magnesium intake for overall health.

Ingredients:

>   - 1/2 cup of magnesium chloride flakes
>
>   - 1/3 cup of distilled water
>
>   - 2 tablespoons of 99.9% pure DMSO
>
>   - 1/4 cup of aloe vera gel (to soothe and hydrate the skin)
>
>   - Glass mixing bowl
>
>   - Glass or plastic storage container with a lid

Portions: Yields approximately 1 cup of magnesium supplement gel.

Step-by-Step Instructions:

>   1. Heat the distilled water in a small saucepan until it is hot but not boiling.
>
>   2. Place the magnesium chloride flakes into the glass mixing bowl.
>
>   3. Pour the hot water over the magnesium chloride flakes, stirring continuously with a non-metallic spoon until the flakes are completely dissolved.
>
>   4. Allow the magnesium solution to cool to room temperature.
>
>   5. Once cooled, add 2 tablespoons of 99.9% pure DMSO to the magnesium solution. Mix thoroughly to ensure the DMSO is well integrated.
>
>   6. Add 1/4 cup of aloe vera gel to the mixture. Stir until the aloe vera gel is fully incorporated and the mixture has a smooth, gel-like consistency.
>
>   7. Transfer the magnesium supplement gel into a glass or plastic storage container. Seal the container tightly to prevent evaporation.

Application Mode:

- Apply a small amount of the magnesium supplement gel to areas of the body experiencing muscle soreness or cramps, gently massaging into the skin until fully absorbed.

- Use up to twice daily, focusing on areas in need of relief or where magnesium absorption is desired.

Precautions:

- Conduct a patch test on a small area of skin before widespread use to ensure no allergic reaction occurs.

- Avoid contact with eyes, mucous membranes, and open wounds.

- Use the gel in a well-ventilated area to minimize inhalation of DMSO fumes.

- Consult with a healthcare professional before using this gel, especially if you are pregnant, nursing, or have a medical condition.

Additional Tips:

- Store the magnesium supplement gel in a cool, dark place to maintain its efficacy. Refrigeration is recommended but not necessary.

- If the gel causes any irritation or discomfort, reduce the frequency of application or discontinue use and consult a healthcare professional.

- For enhanced benefits, consider applying the gel after a warm shower or bath when the skin is more permeable to increase magnesium absorption.

DMSO and Zinc Oxide Cream

Objective: To formulate a skin-soothing cream that utilizes the anti-inflammatory properties of zinc oxide, enhanced with the deep tissue penetration capabilities of DMSO, for effective skin protection and healing.

Benefits: This cream combines the protective and healing properties of zinc oxide, widely recognized for its ability to soothe skin irritations, rashes, and burns, with DMSO's ability to enhance absorption into the skin. It's designed to provide a barrier against irritants while promoting faster healing of the skin.

Ingredients:

- 2 tablespoons of 99.9% pure DMSO

- 1/4 cup of zinc oxide powder

- 1/2 cup of shea butter (as a base)

- 2 tablespoons of coconut oil (to moisturize)

- 1 tablespoon of beeswax (to thicken the cream)

- 10 drops of lavender essential oil (optional, for scent and additional skin benefits)

- Double boiler

- Glass or metal storage container with a lid

Portions: Yields approximately 8 ounces of cream.

Step-by-Step Instructions:

1. Begin by melting the shea butter, coconut oil, and beeswax together in a double boiler over medium heat. Stir continuously until all ingredients are melted and well combined.

2. Remove the mixture from heat and allow it to cool slightly, but not solidify. This ensures the DMSO and zinc oxide can be mixed in effectively without degrading their properties.

3. Gradually add 2 tablespoons of 99.9% pure DMSO to the mixture, stirring thoroughly to ensure it's evenly distributed throughout the cream.

4. Slowly sift in 1/4 cup of zinc oxide powder to the mixture, stirring continuously to prevent clumping and ensure a smooth consistency.

5. If using, add 10 drops of lavender essential oil to the mixture for additional skin healing benefits and a pleasant scent. Stir well to incorporate.

6. Once all ingredients are fully mixed and the cream has a smooth consistency, carefully pour the mixture into a glass or metal storage container. Allow the cream to cool and solidify at room temperature.

7. Seal the container with a lid to prevent contamination and preserve the cream's efficacy.

Application Mode:

- Clean and dry the affected area of skin before application.

- Using clean fingers or a spatula, apply a small amount of the DMSO and Zinc Oxide Cream to the skin.

- Gently massage the cream into the skin until it is fully absorbed, focusing on areas that need protection or healing.

- Apply the cream 2-3 times daily, or as needed, to maintain skin protection and promote healing.

Precautions:

- Conduct a patch test on a small area of skin before using extensively, especially if you have sensitive skin, to ensure no adverse reaction occurs.

- Avoid contact with eyes, mucous membranes, and open wounds.

- Use the cream in a well-ventilated area to minimize inhalation of DMSO fumes.

- Consult with a healthcare professional before using this cream if you are pregnant, nursing, or have a medical condition.

Additional Tips:

- Store the cream in a cool, dark place to maintain its potency. Refrigeration is not necessary but can provide a cooling effect upon application.

- If the cream is too thick or hard to spread, gently warm the container in your hands before use.

- For enhanced skin healing, maintain a balanced diet rich in vitamins and minerals to support the body's natural healing processes.

11.2: DMSO WITH HERBAL REMEDIES & OILS

When considering the integration of **DMSO** with **herbal remedies and essential oils**, it's crucial to understand the specific properties and benefits of each herb and oil to tailor the treatment to individual needs effectively. For instance, **lavender oil** is renowned for its calming and anti-inflammatory properties, making it an excellent choice for blends aimed at reducing anxiety or skin inflammation. To create a **DMSO and lavender oil blend**, start by mixing 1 part of high-quality, therapeutic-grade lavender essential oil with 9 parts of 99% pure DMSO. This ratio ensures the solution is potent yet safe for topical application, particularly useful for areas affected by stress-induced skin conditions or minor burns.

Similarly, **tea tree oil**, known for its antimicrobial and antiseptic qualities, can be combined with DMSO to enhance its penetration and efficacy in treating acne or fungal infections. A blend of 2 parts tea tree oil to 8 parts DMSO can be applied directly to the affected area using a cotton swab, avoiding the surrounding healthy skin to prevent irritation. It's important to conduct a patch test prior to full application to ensure no adverse reactions occur.

For those dealing with joint pain or arthritis, incorporating **ginger oil** into a DMSO blend can offer significant relief. Ginger oil's anti-inflammatory and analgesic properties, when enhanced by DMSO's deep tissue penetration, can reduce pain and improve mobility. Mixing 3 parts ginger oil with 7 parts DMSO creates a powerful rub that can be massaged into sore joints and muscles twice daily. Wearing gloves during application prevents the DMSO from carrying any unintended substances through the skin and allows for a more comfortable application process.

Peppermint oil, with its cooling sensation and natural analgesic effects, can be blended with DMSO for a soothing remedy for headaches or muscle spasms. A mixture of 1 part peppermint oil to 9 parts DMSO, applied to the temples, neck, or affected muscles, provides rapid relief. The cooling effect of peppermint oil is immediately felt, while the DMSO works to deliver the oil's analgesic properties deeper into the tissues.

Creating a **DMSO and chamomile oil blend** can be particularly beneficial for skin conditions like eczema or psoriasis. Chamomile oil's anti-inflammatory and healing properties, combined with DMSO, can soothe the skin and accelerate healing. A gentle blend of 1 part chamomile oil to 9 parts DMSO can be applied to the affected areas with a soft brush, ensuring the blend is evenly distributed and absorbed.

For each of these blends, using pharmaceutical-grade DMSO is imperative to ensure purity and safety. Additionally, sourcing organic, therapeutic-grade essential oils guarantees the absence of any synthetic additives that could react unfavorably with DMSO. The specific ratios provided here are starting points; adjustments may be necessary based on individual skin sensitivity and the severity of the condition being treated. Regular monitoring of the skin's response to these blends is crucial, and any signs of irritation or adverse reaction should prompt immediate discontinuation of use. Consulting with a healthcare professional before beginning any new treatment regimen is always recommended, especially for individuals with pre-existing conditions or those taking other medications.

11.2.1: DMSO Herbal Remedy Recipes

DMSO and Sage Oil Infusion

Objective: To create a therapeutic infusion using DMSO and sage oil, designed to alleviate joint pain and reduce inflammation through the natural healing properties of sage and the enhanced penetration of DMSO.

Benefits: This infusion harnesses the anti-inflammatory and antioxidant properties of sage oil, combined with the deep tissue penetration capabilities of DMSO, to provide relief from joint pain, muscle soreness, and inflammation.

Ingredients:

- 2 tablespoons of 99.9% pure DMSO

- 1/4 cup of sage essential oil

- 1/2 cup of olive oil (as a carrier oil)

- Glass jar with a tight-fitting lid

Portions: Yields approximately 3/4 cup of DMSO and Sage Oil Infusion.

Step-by-Step Instructions:

1. In a clean, dry glass jar, combine 1/4 cup of sage essential oil with 1/2 cup of olive oil. The olive oil acts as a carrier, diluting the sage essential oil to a safe concentration for skin application.

2. Add 2 tablespoons of 99.9% pure DMSO to the oil mixture. Use a non-metallic stirrer to mix the ingredients thoroughly until the DMSO is fully integrated with the oils. The DMSO will not only enhance the penetration of the sage oil into the skin but also contribute to the anti-inflammatory and pain-relieving effects.

3. Seal the jar tightly with its lid to prevent any evaporation or contamination of the infusion.

4. Store the jar in a cool, dark place for 24 hours to allow the ingredients to infuse fully. Gently shake the jar a few times during this period to ensure the ingredients are well combined.

Application Mode:

- Shake the jar gently before each use to ensure the infusion is well mixed.

- Apply a small amount of the DMSO and Sage Oil Infusion to the affected area, using clean fingers or a cotton pad.

- Gently massage the infusion into the skin in a circular motion until it is fully absorbed. Focus on areas with joint pain, muscle soreness, or inflammation.

- Use up to twice daily, preferably once in the morning to alleviate stiffness and once in the evening for overnight relief.

Precautions:

- Conduct a patch test on a small, inconspicuous area of skin before widespread use to ensure no allergic reaction occurs.

- Avoid contact with eyes, mucous membranes, and open wounds.

- Use the infusion in a well-ventilated area to minimize inhalation of DMSO fumes.

- Consult with a healthcare professional before using this infusion, especially if you are pregnant, nursing, or have a medical condition.

Additional Tips:

- Store the infusion in a cool, dark place to maintain its potency. Refrigeration is not necessary but can extend the shelf life.

- If the scent of sage is too strong, the amount of sage essential oil can be adjusted according to personal preference. However, do not alter the recommended amount of DMSO.

- For enhanced benefits, consider wrapping the treated area with a warm cloth after application to increase absorption and provide additional relief.

DMSO and Fennel Seed Gel

Objective: To craft a therapeutic gel using DMSO and fennel seeds, designed to alleviate digestive discomfort and bloating through topical application.

Benefits: This gel combines the anti-inflammatory and antispasmodic properties of fennel seeds with the deep tissue penetration of DMSO, offering relief from digestive issues such as bloating, gas, and cramps.

Ingredients:

> - 2 tablespoons of fennel seeds
>
> - 1 cup of distilled water
>
> - 2 tablespoons of 99.9% pure DMSO
>
> - 1/4 cup of aloe vera gel (to soothe and hydrate the skin)
>
> - Cheesecloth or fine mesh strainer
>
> - Glass mixing bowl
>
> - Glass or plastic storage container with a lid

Portions: Yields approximately 1/2 cup of gel.

Step-by-Step Instructions:

> 1. Begin by boiling 1 cup of distilled water in a small saucepan. Once boiling, add 2 tablespoons of fennel seeds. Reduce the heat and simmer for 10 minutes to create a strong fennel infusion.

> 2. Remove the saucepan from the heat and allow the fennel infusion to cool to room temperature.

> 3. Strain the fennel seeds from the water using cheesecloth or a fine mesh strainer, collecting the infused water in a glass mixing bowl. Press the seeds to extract as much liquid as possible.

> 4. Add 2 tablespoons of 99.9% pure DMSO to the fennel-infused water. Stir thoroughly to ensure the DMSO is fully dissolved.

> 5. Mix in 1/4 cup of aloe vera gel into the DMSO and fennel solution. Stir until the mixture achieves a consistent gel-like texture.

> 6. Transfer the gel into a glass or plastic storage container. Seal the container tightly to prevent evaporation and contamination.

Application Mode:

- Apply a generous amount of the DMSO and Fennel Seed Gel to the abdomen, gently massaging in a circular motion until fully absorbed.

- Use the gel up to twice daily, especially before meals or at times of digestive discomfort.

Precautions:

- Conduct a patch test on a small area of skin before general application to ensure no allergic reaction occurs.

- Avoid contact with eyes, mucous membranes, and open wounds.

- Use the gel in a well-ventilated area to minimize inhalation of DMSO fumes.

- Consult with a healthcare professional before using this gel if you are pregnant, nursing, or have a medical condition, especially related to digestion.

Additional Tips:

- Store the gel in a cool, dark place to maintain its potency. Refrigeration is recommended but not necessary.

- For enhanced digestive support, consider incorporating dietary sources of fennel into your meals, such as adding fennel seeds to salads or drinking fennel tea.

- Ensure to stay hydrated and maintain a balanced diet to support overall digestive health.

Part 4:
Advanced Uses of DMSO

Chapter 12:
Internal Use of DMSO

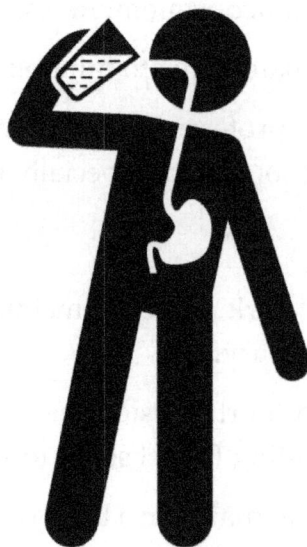

When considering the **internal use of DMSO**, it's paramount to understand the **dosage and concentration** levels that are deemed safe for consumption. The **FDA** has approved DMSO for limited medical conditions, which underscores the importance of adhering to **specific guidelines** when using it internally. A **starting point** for safe internal use is often a **low concentration**, typically around **0.1% to 1%**, which can be gradually increased based on tolerance and under professional supervision. It's crucial to use **pharmaceutical-grade DMSO** as it meets the purity standards required for medical use, ensuring that it's free from contaminants that could be harmful if ingested.

The **method of preparation** involves diluting DMSO in distilled water or another suitable carrier. For instance, mixing 1 ml of 99.9% pharmaceutical-grade DMSO with 99 ml of distilled water would create a 1% DMSO solution. This solution can be taken orally, but it's essential to start with a **small dose** to monitor the body's response. A typical **starting**

dose might be one teaspoon of a 1% DMSO solution per day, gradually increasing to no more than two teaspoons per day, as advised by a healthcare professional.

Monitoring the body's response is critical when ingesting DMSO. Some individuals may experience **side effects**, such as gastrointestinal discomfort, headaches, or dizziness. If any adverse reactions occur, it's advisable to **reduce the dosage** or cease internal use and consult a healthcare provider. Additionally, maintaining **hydration** is important, as DMSO can have diuretic effects.

Interactions with medications and supplements should also be considered. DMSO can enhance the absorption of certain substances, potentially leading to **increased effects or toxicity**. Therefore, discussing the use of DMSO with a healthcare provider is crucial, especially for individuals taking **prescription medications**, over-the-counter drugs, or **dietary supplements**.

For those opting for internal use, incorporating **antioxidants** in the diet or as supplements may be beneficial. Antioxidants like **vitamin C**, **vitamin E**, and **selenium** can help counteract any potential oxidative stress caused by DMSO. However, the timing of antioxidant intake should be staggered from DMSO consumption to prevent interference with its action.

Finally, the **duration of internal DMSO use** should be limited to short-term applications, focusing on specific health objectives, and always under the guidance of a healthcare professional. Long-term internal use is not recommended due to the lack of extensive research on its safety profile. Regular **health check-ups** and **laboratory tests** can help monitor the effects of DMSO on the body's overall function and ensure that its use remains within safe parameters.

12.1: ORAL PROTOCOLS FOR SAFE USE

When considering the **oral consumption of DMSO**, it is crucial to ensure that the **pharmaceutical-grade DMSO** is being used. This grade guarantees the highest purity, minimizing the risk of contaminants that could pose health risks when ingested. Begin with a **1% DMSO solution**, which can be prepared by diluting 1 ml of 99.9% pure DMSO in 99 ml of distilled water. This low concentration is essential to minimize potential side effects and allows for the body to adjust to DMSO. The initial dose should be **one teaspoon of the 1% solution daily**, closely monitoring for any adverse reactions such as gastrointestinal discomfort or allergic reactions. If tolerated well, the dosage can be gradually increased, not exceeding **two teaspoons per day**, under the guidance of a healthcare professional.

Hydration plays a pivotal role in mitigating DMSO's diuretic effects, hence, increasing water intake is advised to prevent dehydration. It's also imperative to be aware of DMSO's capacity to enhance the absorption of other compounds. This characteristic can lead to increased potency of medications or supplements being taken concurrently, which could inadvertently elevate their effects to toxic levels. Therefore, a detailed discussion with a healthcare provider about current medications and supplements is necessary to avoid adverse interactions.

Incorporating **antioxidants** such as **vitamin C, vitamin E**, and **selenium** into the diet or as supplements may offer protective benefits against potential oxidative stress induced by DMSO. However, it's important to stagger the intake of these antioxidants and DMSO to prevent any interference with DMSO's therapeutic actions. Given the diuretic effect of DMSO, monitoring for signs of dehydration and maintaining adequate hydration is crucial.

The use of DMSO internally should be approached with caution, emphasizing short-term use directed towards specific health goals. Continuous monitoring by a healthcare professional, including regular health check-ups and laboratory tests, is essential to ensure safety and efficacy. This cautious approach allows for adjustments to the protocol based on the individual's response and emerging scientific evidence.

12.2: BENEFITS AND RISKS OF DMSO INGESTION

The potential benefits of ingesting DMSO are closely tied to its unique properties as a solvent and its ability to penetrate biological membranes, which can facilitate the delivery of certain medications or nutrients directly into the cells. For instance, DMSO's ability to enhance cellular absorption can be leveraged to improve the bioavailability of supplements such as **vitamin C** or **magnesium**, potentially amplifying their health benefits. This characteristic makes DMSO a valuable tool in scenarios where increasing the effectiveness of a treatment or supplement is desired. Moreover, DMSO has been observed to exhibit **anti-inflammatory** effects, which could be beneficial in reducing systemic inflammation, a root cause of numerous chronic diseases. Its antioxidant properties also suggest a role in neutralizing free radicals, thereby offering protection against oxidative stress and contributing to cellular health and longevity.

However, the risks associated with the ingestion of DMSO cannot be overlooked. One of the primary concerns is its potential to carry other substances through the skin and into the bloodstream, which, while beneficial in controlled therapeutic contexts, poses a significant risk if DMSO is contaminated with toxic substances. This underscores the importance of using only pharmaceutical-grade DMSO under the guidance of a healthcare professional. Additionally, the body metabolizes DMSO into **dimethyl sulfide**, a compound that can cause a garlic-like odor in the breath and body excretions, which may be socially uncomfortable for some individuals. More seriously, DMSO's interaction with certain medications raises the risk of enhanced or altered drug effects, potentially leading to toxicity if not carefully managed. Gastrointestinal discomfort, headaches, and allergic reactions are among the reported side effects, emphasizing the need for cautious, informed use.

Given these considerations, the decision to use DMSO internally should be made with careful deliberation and professional oversight. Starting with a low concentration and closely monitoring the body's response allows for the identification of any adverse effects before they become serious. It is also crucial to maintain open communication with a healthcare provider, especially regarding the concurrent use of medications or supplements, to mitigate the risk of harmful interactions. The integration of antioxidants into the regimen may offer protective benefits against potential oxidative stress induced by DMSO, but timing and dosage should be managed to avoid interference with its therapeutic effects. Ultimately, the use of DMSO for internal applications should be approached with a focus on safety, efficacy, and the principle of 'do no harm,' ensuring that the potential benefits outweigh the risks involved.

Chapter 13:
DMSO in Chronic Condition Management

In the realm of chronic condition management, DMSO (dimethyl sulfoxide) emerges as a compelling adjunct therapy, offering a beacon of hope for those grappling with persistent health challenges. Its unique properties, including the ability to penetrate biological membranes and deliver therapeutic agents directly to the cells, make it an invaluable tool in the arsenal against chronic diseases. The application of DMSO in managing conditions such as fibromyalgia, rheumatoid arthritis, and interstitial cystitis demonstrates its versatility and potential to alleviate symptoms and improve quality of life. For individuals battling fibromyalgia, a condition characterized by widespread musculoskeletal pain accompanied by fatigue, sleep, memory, and mood issues, DMSO offers a pathway to relief. By applying a DMSO solution topically to the affected areas, patients may experience a reduction in pain and inflammation, attributed to DMSO's anti-inflammatory and analgesic properties. The protocol involves gently rubbing a DMSO solution—typically ranging from 30% to 70% concentration, diluted in distilled water—onto the skin over the painful regions. Care must be taken to start with a lower concentration to assess skin sensitivity and tolerance, gradually increasing as needed and tolerated.

For those suffering from rheumatoid arthritis, an autoimmune disorder that affects the joints causing pain, swelling, and stiffness, DMSO can be a game-changer. The treatment protocol might include applying a 50% DMSO solution mixed with aloe vera gel to soothe the skin and enhance penetration, directly to the swollen joints. This combination not only targets inflammation but also aids in moisturizing the skin, minimizing the dryness that can accompany DMSO use. It's advisable to apply the mixture twice daily, monitoring for any adverse reactions and adjusting the frequency and concentration accordingly.

Interstitial cystitis, a chronic condition manifesting as bladder pressure, bladder pain, and sometimes pelvic pain, presents another area where DMSO's therapeutic potential shines. Intravesical administration of DMSO, where the solution is directly instilled into the bladder, has shown promise in reducing symptoms and improving the quality of life for affected individuals. This procedure, typically carried out in a clinical setting, involves a healthcare professional introducing a 50% DMSO solution into the bladder via a catheter. Patients may experience relief from pain and urgency after just a few treatments, highlighting DMSO's role as a potent anti-inflammatory agent.

The cornerstone of utilizing DMSO in chronic condition management lies in its ability to modulate inflammation, a common thread linking many chronic diseases. By addressing inflammation at its source, DMSO helps to mitigate the cascading effects that contribute to the symptomatology of these conditions. However, it's imperative to approach DMSO therapy with caution, adhering to recommended guidelines for concentration, application methods, and frequency to avoid potential side effects. Ensuring the use of pharmaceutical-grade DMSO is paramount, as is consulting with a healthcare professional to tailor the therapy to the individual's specific needs and health status.

Beyond these specific conditions, DMSO's utility extends to managing symptoms in other chronic diseases, such as scleroderma, a rare autoimmune disease that leads to hardening and tightening of the skin and connective tissues. In such cases, DMSO's ability to penetrate deep into the tissues can help alleviate the discomfort associated with skin and tissue stiffness. A protocol for scleroderma might involve applying a 50% DMSO solution to the affected areas daily, with careful observation for any skin reactions or improvements in symptoms, adjusting the treatment frequency as necessary.

Moreover, DMSO's antioxidative properties offer potential benefits in the management of oxidative stress-related conditions, such as chronic fatigue syndrome and certain neurological disorders. By neutralizing free radicals, DMSO may help reduce the oxidative damage that contributes to the fatigue and cognitive impairments observed in these conditions. For chronic fatigue syndrome, a topical application of a 30% DMSO solution to areas of pain and inflammation could provide symptomatic relief, enhancing the patient's overall energy levels and quality of life.

In the realm of neurological disorders, particularly those involving nerve pain like trigeminal neuralgia, DMSO's analgesic properties can be leveraged to provide pain relief. A carefully prepared blend of DMSO with anti-inflammatory essential oils, such as lavender or peppermint, applied to the cheek or jaw area, may offer a reduction in nerve pain intensity. This approach underscores the importance of combining DMSO with complementary therapies to maximize its therapeutic benefits.

When integrating DMSO into a chronic condition management plan, it's crucial to maintain a holistic perspective, considering the patient's overall health, lifestyle, and concurrent treatments. This includes evaluating the potential for DMSO to interact with other medications and supplements, as its solvent properties can enhance the absorption and potency of concurrently used substances. A thorough discussion with healthcare professionals about all medications and supplements being taken is essential to avoid unintended interactions and ensure a harmonious and effective treatment regimen.

Additionally, the importance of lifestyle factors such as diet, exercise, and stress management cannot be overstated in managing chronic conditions. Incorporating DMSO therapy into a comprehensive care plan that includes these elements can synergize to improve outcomes. For instance, a diet rich in anti-inflammatory foods may complement DMSO's inflammation-modulating effects, while regular, gentle exercise can help maintain mobility and reduce pain.

Patient education and empowerment are key components of successful chronic condition management with DMSO. Providing individuals with detailed information on how to safely use DMSO, including proper dilution techniques, application methods, and storage, empowers them to take an active role in their care. Encouraging patients to keep a symptom diary can help track the effectiveness of DMSO therapy over time, facilitating adjustments to the treatment plan based on observed outcomes.

Chapter 14:
DMSO for Anti-Aging and Cellular Health

In the quest for anti-aging solutions and optimal cellular health, DMSO (dimethyl sulfoxide) emerges as a potent ally, offering a multifaceted approach to slowing down the aging process and enhancing cellular function. This compound, known for its remarkable ability to penetrate the skin and other biological membranes, delivers therapeutic agents directly to the cells, promoting healing and regeneration at the molecular level. The anti-aging potential of DMSO lies in its antioxidant properties, which play a crucial role in neutralizing free radicals. Free radicals are unstable molecules that can cause damage to cells, proteins, and DNA, contributing to aging and various diseases. By scavenging these harmful molecules, DMSO helps to mitigate oxidative stress, a key factor in the aging process.

Moreover, DMSO's anti-inflammatory capabilities are instrumental in combating chronic inflammation, another hallmark of aging. Chronic inflammation is associated with a wide range of age-related conditions, including arthritis, cardiovascular disease, and neurodegenerative disorders. By reducing inflammation, DMSO aids in preserving the integrity of cells and tissues, thereby supporting their longevity and functionality.

The application of DMSO for anti-aging purposes extends beyond its antioxidant and anti-inflammatory effects. DMSO has been shown to enhance the absorption and efficacy of other anti-aging compounds, such as vitamins, minerals, and herbal extracts. When used in conjunction with these nutrients, DMSO can facilitate their delivery into the cells, amplifying their beneficial effects on skin health, tissue repair, and overall wellness. This synergistic interaction underscores the versatility of DMSO as a component of integrative anti-aging protocols.

To harness the anti-aging benefits of DMSO, it is essential to adopt a targeted approach, focusing on specific areas of concern. For skin rejuvenation, a topical application of DMSO mixed with anti-aging agents like vitamin C, hyaluronic acid, or retinol can improve skin texture, elasticity, and appearance. This combination can help to reduce the visibility of fine lines, wrinkles, and age spots, promoting a more youthful complexion. It is important to start with a low concentration of DMSO to assess skin tolerance and gradually increase it as needed, ensuring optimal results without irritation.

In addition to topical applications, DMSO can be used to enhance the effectiveness of supplements aimed at supporting cellular health and longevity. For instance, mixing

DMSO with antioxidant-rich supplements such as resveratrol, CoQ10, or alpha-lipoic acid can boost their bioavailability and therapeutic impact. This approach not only targets the external signs of aging but also addresses the underlying cellular processes, offering a comprehensive strategy for health and longevity.

As with any therapeutic regimen, the key to success lies in personalization and adherence to safety guidelines. Consulting with a healthcare professional experienced in the use of DMSO is crucial to developing a customized anti-aging protocol that aligns with individual health needs and goals. This ensures the safe and effective use of DMSO, maximizing its potential benefits while minimizing any risks.

For enhancing joint health and flexibility, which often decline with age, DMSO can be applied in a diluted form to areas affected by stiffness or discomfort. This application can provide relief and support mobility, thanks to DMSO's deep penetration and anti-inflammatory properties. Creating a blend of DMSO with essential oils known for their soothing effects, such as lavender or eucalyptus, can further enhance this benefit. It's imperative to ensure that the essential oils are of therapeutic grade and properly diluted to avoid skin irritation.

Incorporating DMSO into a regimen aimed at cognitive health can also be beneficial. The compound's ability to cross the blood-brain barrier means it can deliver neuroprotective compounds directly to the brain. A protocol might include DMSO-enhanced delivery of supplements like Ginkgo Biloba or Omega-3 fatty acids, which have been shown to support brain health and cognitive function. Careful consideration of the timing and dosage is necessary to optimize the benefits while minimizing potential risks, such as irritation or unwanted interactions with other medications.

For systemic anti-aging effects, incorporating DMSO into a daily routine by mixing it with a carrier oil like coconut or jojoba oil and applying it to the skin can help deliver antioxidants and other beneficial compounds throughout the body. This method leverages DMSO's transdermal delivery capabilities to support overall wellness and combat aging from the inside out.

When considering the use of DMSO for anti-aging, it's also important to integrate other health-promoting practices such as a balanced diet rich in antioxidants, regular physical activity, and adequate hydration. These lifestyle factors work synergistically with DMSO to enhance its anti-aging effects and support optimal health.

Monitoring the body's response to DMSO is crucial, as individual reactions can vary. Starting with a small test application and gradually increasing usage allows for the identification of any sensitivities or adverse reactions. Documenting this process can help in adjusting the approach for better results.

Finally, staying informed about the latest research and developments in the field of anti-aging and DMSO use is beneficial. The landscape of health and wellness is continually evolving, and new discoveries could offer additional insights into how DMSO can be used effectively for anti-aging purposes. Engaging with a community of individuals who are also exploring DMSO for health and longevity can provide support, share experiences, and offer practical advice on navigating the complexities of anti-aging therapies.

Conclusion

EMBRACING A NEW PATH TO NATURAL HEALING

In a world dominated by quick fixes and over-the-counter medications, choosing a natural path like DMSO represents a profound shift in how we approach our own health. Embracing DMSO isn't just about trying a new supplement; it's about adopting a philosophy of healing that respects the body's innate wisdom. This path acknowledges that true wellness doesn't always come from suppressing symptoms, but from addressing the root causes of discomfort, pain, and imbalance. By choosing DMSO, you're investing in a holistic approach that works *with* your body rather than against it, tapping into its natural rhythms and resilience.

The journey you've taken through this book has given you a foundation of knowledge and practical skills to use DMSO safely and effectively. You've learned about its unique properties, its scientifically-backed mechanisms, and its profound impact on conditions ranging from chronic pain to inflammation. But this journey goes beyond the technical aspects; it invites you to take a more empowered role in your health. In embracing DMSO, you are also choosing a path of mindfulness, where you tune into your body's responses, adjusting and refining as you go. This dynamic relationship with your own health fosters a deeper awareness of your body's needs and encourages you to take proactive steps that support long-term wellness.

Transitioning to natural healing approaches like DMSO means prioritizing patience and attentiveness, qualities often overlooked in conventional medicine. With DMSO, relief may not always be instantaneous, but it is comprehensive and often transformative. This approach encourages us to be active participants in our health journeys, observing how our bodies respond, learning what works best, and making adjustments to find optimal results. Unlike medications designed to mask symptoms, DMSO helps the body restore itself, and by working alongside it, you foster a greater sense of partnership in your healing journey. This mindful, responsive approach allows you to not only alleviate discomfort but to truly understand and address the origins of your symptoms, setting the stage for sustainable well-being.

Thank you for choosing this path, for trusting in your ability to learn, and for embracing the possibilities of wellness. Here's to a future where knowledge and wellness guide each step—empowering you to live a life of health, balance, and empowerment.

Made in the USA
Las Vegas, NV
06 March 2025